WONDERS IN DEMENTIALAND™

By Suzka

USBN-13: 978-0-692-79524-8

My mother forgot how
she fit in the past. She forgot
how to see into the future.
She only knew of today where
she was able to see all of her self
centered in the middle
of spectacular!

Ah, the wonders I found in Dementialand.

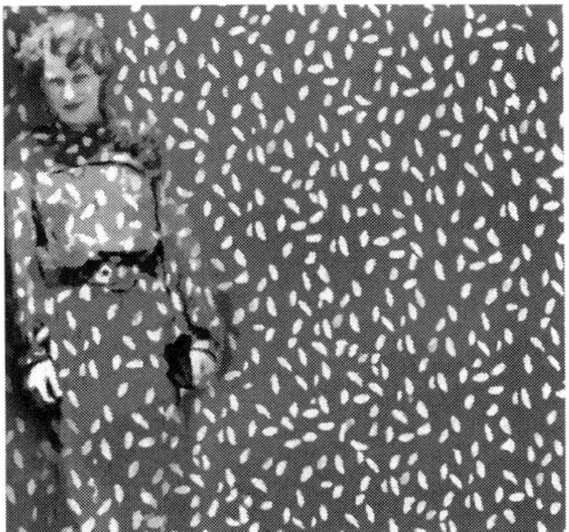

Contents:

Suzka

c.27

Dementia pursued my mother in the nights. Maybe it was when she danced with the gypsies that it had made up its mind that it was going to have her for its own. It would not be easy. My mother had guarded her wits and hid them from us as well as the night's sundown robbers. But dementia carefully thought this through. It knew it had to be patient if it wanted to have its prize in the end.

Dementia hid behind trees on the side of the night's moons and in dark's empty spaces, waiting for its chance. It followed behind quietly and whispered her name. Wherever Violet went she heard its echo.

Violet disappeared more often, sometimes for only a few seconds, other times for an entire day. In some ways, it was as if she was having an affair. She couldn't hide the change that was inside of her – the unfaithfulness to status quo, to the norm, to the structure and temples she had built. I couldn't help but notice her struggling with the unexplainable pandemonium jumping inside of her and the guilt that pushed away its promised happiness. There was a scary freedom that only a new love brings. A wide freedom so big and so loud it disturbs and whacks everything in its path. Was my mother holding on to a secret, afraid she might get caught, worried that her new lover would call for her impulsively at any time? How could anyone resist a new love's passion? I found myself obsessed in wandering curiosity. Where does she go when she leaves me?

[I gave myself no choice
but to think like a painter.
It kept me sane.
My friend Gulley Jimson
once told me that even the
worst artist that ever was,
a cross-eyed mental deficient
with the shakes in both hands,
about to paint the first stroke,
looks at the blank canvas
as an adventure.

This was a fresh canvas.]

Suzka

It all started in December. My mother drove to church that day. Her bloody eye would have been a shallow excuse to the Gods who appreciated the sacrifices of true martyrs. With one hand, she used a full roll of paper towels and pressed it firmly over her bruises to stop the bleeding; her other hand gripped the steering wheel. When she got close enough to the church property, she made a quick turn and rolled over the curb without notice. The God's mercifully bumper stopped her at the cement steps at the building's entrance.

Violet put everything in park, got out and limped into the church with the heavy velvet syllables of Latin in her steps. Syllables she had sung to herself when she was alone in her kitchen.

Her eyelids were fat and stuffy. The right eyeball lost all its white. A rage of purple-like color filled its socket. Blood had been stuck around the cut on her forehead. From her shoulders down, other than the perfumed air of Campho-Phenique that followed her, Violet was girdled, nylon'ed, tucked and wearing her Sergio Rossi high heels like any other morning.

The statue'd saints and virgins saw Violet walk into the church and stopped their solemnness to look at their newest martyr. One lady still settling herself in the pew saw Violet and screamed. The scream echoed throughout the church, changing the holy deadness in the air.

"Violet, Vwaht on God's earth happen to you?"

[Everyone who was not my sister
called my mother Violet]

A crowd of ladies circled their attentions to Violet's bleeding wound. A few ladies dug in their pockets and purses for Kleenex to wipe the blood that had now dripped down her neck and made a line around the collar of her white blouse.

Other women beat their breasts trying to remember the patron saint for bad cuts. Violet would know but no one would ask.

"Violet, what happened? You're bleeding?" Ellie, a close friend, always had a calm way when talking to Violet, in any emergency.

"Violet, tell me what happened to you?"

The rank of service reversed its order. The ladies were now the apostles of the moment. The little priest with his purple cape floated down the altar's steps and melted into the back of the fold.

One of the ladies shouted, "She lookca like she'za been mugga."

Another voice from somewhere, "Ooh my Lawd. Jesu, she been mugg!"

The word mugged was repeated and passed around in soft whispers within the ladies as if they were fresh baked anise cookies.

The ladies pulled Violet to the closest pew and set her down.

"No. No. No. I put campho on it. I'm ok."

Ellie took Violet's hand and looked closer at the wound.

"But Violet, you're bleeding, you're hurt. You need to go to the hospital."

One of the ladies turned her head around and repeated the words she heard for the others in the back.

“They saza she needsa to go to the hospitaw.”

Another added with sincere but weightless assistance,"My daughter-in-law sister work at hospita. I call her. Yes?" said another patron.

From the back, "Someone call 911."

"I'm fine. No. No. No. If I need to go, I will drive myself to the hospital."

No one really listened or paid much attention to Violet at this point.

"Call 911. Someone call 911 right now."

From the side, the little priest solemnly shoved his words between the ladies running chatter. "I will call 911 from the office."

[I could go on, which is exactly what I intend on doing but first I must prepare you – this story has its own reality, and its own truthfulness based on my memory of events that legitimately have no rightness or wrongness to them.

I guess this is the best place to start.
It was in early December…]

*

"Suzka, this is Ellie from the church. I hate to wake you at his hour, but..."

It was 6:27, the early 6:27 in California. The phone rang five times. Ellie's voice came into the studio by itself after traveling over two thousand miles. It was unlike Ellie to call so God awful early in the morning. She was fully aware of my late-into- the-night creative lifestyle. She never called me before noon.

"... your mom had an accident. She told us that she fell in the bathroom and hit her head against the counter. She has quite a bruise on her eye. She came to morning Mass and even the priest stopped the service and went to your mother to see if she was ok. The pastor called 911 and an ambulance took her to Loyola Hospital. Maybe you should fly in as soon as you can."

Ellie was my mother's close friend. She was three decades younger and eight inches taller. Her plain looks changed to adorable when she smiled and laughed. She had easy straight brown hair, cut short, one length except for her bangs that stood fidgeting over her eyebrows like children in a church choir. She often wore flat rubber sole shoes. Ellie and my mother met in church, both were in the choir.

Ellie watched out for my mother, especially in the past year. My mother was somewhat a bit more scattered than usual. Ellie would visit her daily; help her with the mail, separating the junk mail from the second-noticed bills. And she was by my mother's side throughout the year looking for the valuables and the not-so-valuables that were stolen in the middle of the night by persons unknown.

There was a special bond of trust and respect between them. It is sometimes difficult for people of my mother's generation and age to put trust in anyone. Ellie was special. I depended on her and trusted her guidance.

Ellie lived only a few blocks from my mother's home. I lived six states away.

*

Buried under stacks of moving pad blankets, I looked up at my bangs blowing in the cold draft from the rollup door. I tried to piece together what Ellie was saying but Ellie's voice was so sedative, even when she delivered bad news, one couldn't help but feel a fuzzy comfortableness in the worst parts. She was good in that way.

Ellie took me through the steps of the morning. The words cradled my body and rocked me very close to sleep.

I was familiar with my mother's morning routine. That helped my head avoid being tasked with the details. For years, in the morning, every morning, my mother, my mother's mother and her mother had covered their heads with cotton babushkas, lace mantillas or rain bonnets and would walk to church in all weather conditions. They walked quickly, as if the priest, the other church ladies and Jesus himself were waiting for their arrival before the Mass could begin.

The face of the church was old, the women with babushkas and boned fingers were old and the spoken language was Latin old. Slovakian whispers filled in the gaps.

[I never thought my mother religious.
Her natural makeup was more theatrical,
more dramatic – where else could her talents
be more nurtured and appreciated
than in the theater of Catholicism.]

When I was very little, I asked my grandmother why she went to church so much.

"We go to church to ask for forgiveness for our sins."

"What sins?" I'd ask.

"The bad tings the devil makes us do."

"The devil don't mess with me. I would spit in his face and kick him real hard in the shins if he even tries messin' with me. No granma, I know for sure I don't have no devil's sins."

"Yes you do. Everyone has sins."

"I don't think so. Stella told me there's no such thing like sins. Stella may be young, maybe an inch younger than me, but she's real smart. She knows things, Granma."

"Don't talk silly. If there was no sin, there would be no hell. You don't talk to that Stella girl no more."

[We were so Catholic back then.]

This particular morning started as usual. A small quiet group of women entered the church. Their fingers blindly dove into the holy water font then jumped out crossing themselves with its blessings. The women were scattered and isolated in pews. A few shared their space with likenesses to themselves.

They pulled rosaries out from deep pockets; rosaries tangled in Kleenex and small sticky wrapped candies. They prayed in separate dialects, the prayers of the rosary. The air was filled with the soft hisses, sounds of petition, postulation, absolution and forgiveness. Some secretly begged the Madonna to protect their married sons and daughters from their husband or wife's ways. In the yellow light their mouths moved slowly.

The servicing priest with curly colored-black hair dressed himself in the vestibule, a small room in back of the altar filled with ceremonial silks. When he was fully decorated for mass, he walked out to the altar, spread his arms wide like they were the purple wings of a sainted angel and began the morning prayers in front of the small turnout. His voice was always slow and melodic as if he was anointed in a waterless pool of forgotten grace.

The altar table was pristine with white lace and two candles. At his side were two altar boys struggling to stay awake, tightened their teeth, holding in a yawn.

At home Violet hurried herself in getting dressed.

She would miss the first twenty prayers of the rosary.

*

Thirty minutes earlier, Violet's hands had pushed the last loose hairs back into her French twist, then heavily spraying everything to its place. Leaning over the counter, she bent closer into the mirror and squinted at the reflected image - a woman with age wrapped in a chenille flowered robe.

Violet occupied the lower portion of the glass. Yellow wallpaper with tiny roses filled in the top parts. A cross of a tortured man, powdered in the bathroom's airborne talc, hung in the mirror's upper corner looking down at Violet. Not reflected, not part of the reversed appearances of things was a postcard taped on the mirror above the lotions. The post card was dated and taped at its corners. It was sent to her from the oldest of her three daughters who years ago moved under the pictured palm trees. All her daughters live with the palm trees. Violet lives alone in Chicago

As Violet stepped back, the tufted rug beneath her grabbed the heel of her Italian shoe and wouldn't let go. The mirror was soundless. It tried to warn her but her body dropped quickly.

Her head hit the corner of the counter hard. A string of pearls rolled down and latched itself on the cabinet's knob and snapped. Blood splashed out and hit the wall. Pearls left their string and fell into the red sea.

*

Ellie's voice continued telling me about the accident.

"Suzka, I would have waited to call you, but I thought you should know right away so you can make flight arrangements. I am sure the hospital will keep her for a couple of days. Call me when you get to the house."

"Thank you Ellie. I'll check the flights."

I slithered out of my bed slowly and poured my feet into my UGGs. It was terribly cold in the warehouse. I covered my body with a heavy long bathrobe that once belonged to my father. I loved that robe. It was old, worn and had paint on it like every other piece of clothing I owned. I shuffled toward the bathroom meandering through a maze of wet, damp paintings that filled the floor.

I took a quick shower, a brush to the teeth, bungeed my hair to the top of my head and UGG'ed myself to the kitchen island percolator. Coffee first before any decisions were to be made.

As I waited for the pot to stop its perk'ing, I looked over last night's work, which was only a few hours old. I tried to look at the canvases but they were all blurred in with my thoughts.

It's just a bruise.

I kept thinking, it's just a bruise.

I thought to throw-up.

Stage One

SYMPTOMS

No visible signs of dementia

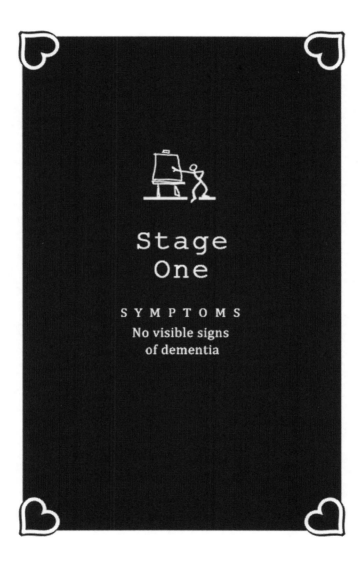

1.
THE JUNK MAN

It was god-awful damp outside. The night was leaning on the late side of dark. Only two streetlights worked on my end of the row and both were quite nervous. One was rather shy with its light and the other stuttered. The fog tried to help the lights by spreading its fluorescent-ness a bit further like water on a paper towel. But all the fog seemed to be good at was slobbering over my duffel bag and my one carry-on.

The bags and I waited outside my painting studio, a cinder block warehouse. Everything was locked up. All my paints inside had their lids hammered down. A few stubborn brushes were soaking in a cut down milk carton resting on the utility sink in the back.

I had called ahead for a taxi and been waiting for what seemed like hours but only seven minutes actually passed. My hands were damp. I was anxious. I could not stop wondering when I would be returning to California, back to my studio, back to painting. My return ticket said three weeks: a generous yet serious amount of time, I thought.

I was fully clothed in the California to Chicago winter-ware. The white cotton t-shirt under a zippered wool vest, a thick buttoned-up cardigan and my black leather bomber jacket; also two cotton skirts, one on top of the other and my signature black tights with the UGGs. I was bed warm and ready for Chicago's December weather.

Twenty minutes already passed. I was restless and weighted in thoughts. The fog began to clear a path for the real morning to appear.

My eyes focused on a neighbor man on the other side of the street who walked out of his house with a steaming mug in his hand. His other hand flicked a lighter's flame close to a fat cigar that was clamped down by his teeth. He stood under a tarred overhang until his cigar was properly lit. His framed house was white and cluttered with junk - treasures rusting in their later years blocked any respectable view. A short picket fence tried to keep his everything contained in a small area about eight feet from the building. From the street you could see old rusty grills, torn lawn chairs and metal injured roosters. There were buggies, wood benches, old Coca-Cola signs and brass monkeys. A screen door rested upright on the side of his house, unattached to its door. Two or three bulging five-gallon bags of dented Budweiser cans filled in the empty spaces.

The neighbor appeared to be a collector of sorts, an entrepreneurial junk man who wore white t-shirts and loose above the ankle jeans held up by thick red suspenders. His hair on the top of his head was sparse, cut short and cropped, his mustache dark, full and bushy. I never formally met the man, I only known of him as *the junk man*.

The junk man looked at me as if he was trying to make out what I was doing standing there in the wet fog, outside my studio, bundled and bagged. He appeared curious but not very interested. He moved around his collection. I stared and thought very carefully - thoughts I preferred not to have but my mind was thinking of alternatives to a possible desperate situation. I needed to get to the airport.

My stare moved from the junk man to a beat up blue Chrysler at the edge of his property under the stuttering lamppost. My head told me it was his car. The car's vinyl top was torn to shreds with a thousand ripped edges rolling over each other. The engine's hood had lost its manufactured color and had a large circle of rust in its center. I squinted a bit hoping my eyes would get a clearer picture into the car's contents. Heavy smoke-stained windows prevented any viewing. It was as if I were yards away from a closed casket at a funeral.

The airport was just a few miles away. Time was moving quickly. Its big hand was pushing the fog aside, making room for clear skies to take over the morning. All the airplanes waited patiently for the skies to tell them they were cleared for takeoff.

Ok. Ok. Ok. I surrendered to the circumstances. An urgency pushed me from behind, shoving me closer to the inevitable. My mouth struggled to lift my face with intentions on creating a cordial smile. I walked to the other side of street and stopped in front of the junk man's property and spoke.

"I'm in a bit of a jam. I need to get to the airport quick but my taxi is..."

My eyes left the junk man and ran up and down the street looking for some reason to stop what I was about to ask. "...well I don't know where in the hell that damn taxi is but it sure isn't here and I need to catch a flight. Do you think, I mean... do you think it is possible, since it doesn't look like you're going anywhere... at the moment, not that I'm assuming you don't have places to go... I mean..."

The junk man pulled the cigar out of his mouth and spoke.

"Spit it out girl. You're making my cigar nervous."

"Do you think you can you drive me to the airport? I'll buy you a case of Budweiser for your trouble."

He swaggered out of his front yard toward the gate and rested his steaming coffee on the ledge of the short picket fence and dug into his pockets fishing out a set of keys and walked to his car. He didn't say yes, he didn't say no. I reluctantly followed hoping I was not going to be that night's local news story: Gifted Artist's Body Parts Found Stuffed in Budweiser Garbage bags.

"Get in. I like cans not the bottles. Remember that. Don't like bottles."

The junk man opened the passenger door. Papers and plastic bottles fell out. He shoved the loose pile of remaining rubble to one side and made just enough room for me to sit. I slid in and balanced my feet on a floor where there were more plastic bottles, pipe tubing, metal scraps, candy wrappers and old receipts. The junk man squished my duffel and carry-on in the back and off we went.

Nothing was said at first. Normal chitchat lost its hospitality somewhere in the garbage.

"So what do you do in that warehouse all by yourself. I can't help but notice there's not a lot of activity goin' on over there. Not a lot of people goin' in and out. Are you one of those recluse types?"

I never heard him speak before. His quick edgy tone matched the swagger, the cigar, the junk and the bulging bags of Budweiser cans in his yard.

"Whadaya' mean? People go in and out all the time." I repeated those defensive words with a more spunky tone of assurance, "People visit me all the time, mostly late at night... you know, the middle of the night... probably when you're asleep." I felt that sassy response smack me in the head. *Why did I say that?*

"Middle of the night, huh?" He rested his arm out the window and twirled his cigar around his grin. He grinned as if I just served him a plate of barbecued ribs. Mine.

I tightened my parameters and avoided resting into the Chrysler. Casually I turned my head and looked out the filmed windows. Wipers dragged themselves across the windshield. My nose was uncomfortable and cautious. I took tiny breaths in an attempt to strip the air from its full flavor. Thank God the airport was only eight miles away.

When we got close to the terminals curb, I opened the door before the car stopped moving and extended my hand. "Thank you."

The junk man's hand for shaking twisted his cigar out of his mouth.

"Remember, cans not bottles."

"Yea... I won't forget."

Slam.

< UNITED AIRLINES >
FLIGHT: #6346 Fri Dec 2
DEPART: California at 5:45 AM
ARRIVE: Chicago at 6:15 PM
RETURN: Jan 17

2.
CALIFORNIA TO CHICAGO

There are places in the world where no one lives, no one belongs and no one is welcome to stay for any extended length of time. They are located in-between countries, between worlds and time zones and are primarily used as transfer centers for millions of traveling migrants. The migrants fly around in pod-like spacecrafts. When their craft lands at one of these places formally identified as airports, an accordion striped of its song expands out to meet the pod. As the pod opens its doors, the accordion then sucks out the traveling migrants from the pod and spits them out into a terminal. I was one of the airport's migrants with a RedEye classification.

*

I navigated my way through the crowd of wrinkled travelers. The slow shuffle reserved for citizens of the Americas at the Tijuana border. It was late and cold. The terminal sign outside the accordion walkway read C31, the furthest gate from the airport's exit. The terminal's clock winked the next minute at 4:12am. I lusted for coffee but the terminal at four twelve was an iridescent ghost town lined with a string of stores covered by corsets of stretched metal. Their neon faces were done. The last call for alcohol, the last 'coffee dripping' was hours ago. Everything was closed.

I followed a large man, carrying a sleeping child just a few bodies in front of me. The child's fist was tightly wound in string. The string knotted itself securely and then went high in the air to a yellow balloon with a wide smile - the same balloon I saw rows in front of where I was sitting earlier on the plane. I remember thinking that the balloon was irritatingly alert and happy for a Redeye flight. With his free hand, the man dragged a carry-on luggage behind him. I followed behind the luggage.

At the end of the corseted stores, past the moving floors, through the neon'ed tunnel was a large baggage-claim area. On one side was a long line of glass doors. The doors worked for the airport. They wore alphabet hats and opened themselves to any travelers passing by. No one could live in the airport world. The doors' job was to entice passing bodies and push them out of the building, throwing them back into the real world. No one had a choice and there were no exceptions. The terminal already had a number of ghosts – previous travelers who refused to leave. They were eventually captured and stuffed in unclaimed baggage. Their families were never notified.

On the opposite side, carousals carried the Samonsites, the Duffels, Briggs & Riley, Tumi and the Louie Vuittons. My bag fell into the carrousel first. Luck. I trudged out of the terminal. The doors behind me turned their backs and folded themselves tightly, sealing the airport world shut.

It was snowing hard. It should have been dark but the snow's white with the moon's help lightened the night. The cold slapped my face and made my eyelids jump and twitch. I was careful to take in just enough of the arctic air that a body required. My nose pushed out the unused and steamed a tiny vapor cloud into the thin air.

[31 inches of snow
fell in Chicago that winter]

I walked to the curb where the limos, taxies and hotel vans picked up their fared travelers. My boots left an impression behind that I had arrived. Layers of clothing protected my skin from freezer burn. My arms pushed up into my jacket, my hands squished together the bottom of the sleeves. I forgot my gloves. I remembered to bring several pairs of sunglasses but not a single pair of gloves.

On a small sheet of paper, tucked in my UGGs, numbers were written - license plate numbers given to me by the limo-cab service. The man driving these numbers would take me to my mother's house.

I squeezed two fingers out from my coat's sleeve and retrieved the paper from my warm UGGs. I hoped the numbers would match Jaidee's limo. He had picked me up from the airport several times. There was an odd bond between us - an enchanting connection that was warm and mysteriously safe in the limo containment. His words were large and never cluttered with worldly drama.

I bounced up and down and swayed back and forth to prevent freezing while keeping my eyes focused in squinting on the unfocused. The snow glazed the limos, cabs and buses. The yellows and blacks were wet and shiny. Round, wiggly lines of color followed the cars from behind. Goose downed people standing around me waved randomly at any car that passed them in hope of being recognized.

The paper stuck loosely between my numb fingers. The numbers 311LVY4 bled, the snow made everything on the paper ooze except for the parts with dried paint. Those smudges of color stood strong. God I love paint. Before I finished my thought about the resilience of paint to the snow, a long black wet limo stopped a few feet away from me at the curb.

Jaidee jumped out quickly and ran around the limo toward me.

"Miz Suzka, I am sorry to be late for your arrival. Are you ok?"

I hardly recognized Jaidee. In the past he would pick me up in a simple black sedan but this time, he was driving the real thing – a long and shiny slick Lincoln with tinted windows.

"Jaidee, is that you? Jesus-Louise, this is pretty fancy. Did you get promoted? And you're wearing a fancy suit jacket, my God, you are lookin' good man."

"It is wicked out here. Let me take your bags. Hurry. Geet in dee car. I put dee heat on very high, to dee max, when I got dee call that your plane is land."

He took my dampened duffel and wheeled my carry-on to the back of the limo.

"You are such a sweetheart." I jumped in quickly and cold-slammed the door. It was exceptionally warm inside and smelled of Jasmine. Not the real Jasmine of course, but I was just as pleased with the processed scent. A soft black couch extended the full length of the limo, which could have easily sat five people. On the other side, was a movie screen and a mini-bar with cut crystal glasses. The ceiling had blue neon lights that wiggled in wavy lines on each side and tiny white stars in the middle that looked as if they were miles away on an exotic island looking up at a summer's sky.

The limo bounced when Jaidee slammed shut the trunk's lid. He moved quickly in the snow's slush and jumped into the driver's side of the car. His hair was covered with white. In seconds the white went away leaving wet cornrow-braided patterns of curves and swirls that gave his head a distinctive shape.

Jaidee blew warm air into his cupped hands. The warmth pushed the chills down his body. He shook.

"Soon you will be toasty warm." He told me.

It was snowing hard. Jaidee moved into the traffic and drove straight into the white air. It was the first snow of the season; the top inches fresh and clean, giving Chicagoans a good impression of winter before the streets stir it up like dirty flour. The white filled the highway wall-to-wall. The road changed and glazed itself as big trucks of salt were grinding the crystals and flavoring the streets. The windshield's rubber wipers squeaked and swayed back and forth, sassy-like, pushing the winter to the side.

I started at the farthest back of the limo, sitting on the soft leather couch for the full-expanded experience but soon moved to the front, closer to Jaidee.

"Jaidee, where's your coat? That frickin' little jacket you're wearing is useless in this freezing cold. Handsome but useless."

"I just dropped off dee mayor's daw'ter. Dat is why tonight I'm driving dee long limo. I wanted to look most professional. I will pick her up in dee ceetee after I take you to your maw'ter's home. Do you like dee auto?"

"I'm not sure - too glitzy for me. I'm expecting a game show host to pop out from somewhere."

I bent over and looked at the line of floor lights under the seat. When I sat back up I met Jaidee's smile in the windshield's mirror. His perfectly lined white teeth filled the reflecting glass.

"I is surprised to see you back so soon."

"I know." My response lost itself in continuing.

Jaidee had picked me up from the airport a number of times. During my last visit he told me that his mother was very ill. A stroke.

"How is your mother, Jaidee?"

"She tiz doing much betta."

"That's good. That's real good." She lived in New Guinea.

Jaidee watched me in his rear view mirror. I caught his looking several times as if he was trying to make out what was different in this return visit. I was never good at deceiving anyone. And I never improved on it. I always relied on my charm and the inspiration of the moment to authenticate my intentions.

'And how iz you Miz Suzka?"

"I'm fine, Jaidee. Just less chatty... tired I guess."

I went into myself and pulled down a curtain with thoughts. He respected my silence and my discomfort in continuing the conversation.

[Jaidee picked me up from the airport
five times just in that past year.
We became close friends.)

My head was filled with daughter's chatter. I was part of those cutout families who prepared the children they made for this very moment. From birth, children are contracted with a scenario already set in place and passed on through generations. Heavy rosaries hung around mothers' necks - gifts from their mothers that they will pass on to their daughters. The string of crystal beads tightening, choking daughters with guilt and obligation. Branded lots of tradition scramble around bumping into each other. They seem to be growing willy-nilly to places where panic and the very worst scenarios survived by sucking the blood from daughtering artists.

I looked down at the dried paint on my hands. There was Terra-Rose, Gold, Indigo and Hooker Green, colors from 'Salinas Landscape Stanzas' – the painting I was working on last night. It was one of my best paintings and now hanging on the back wall in my studio. I always felt warm, centered and somewhat grounded when my hands were spotted with paint that survived its washing.

Picking the dry paint off my hands was an indulging and warming distraction. I first peeled away the dry paint stuck under the nail parts. Specs of color fell onto my lap and scattered across my skirt posing as creations of Seurat and Jackson Pollack. Were they the artists who were sent to deliver the contract - the daughter's contract regarding guardianship?

There was no turning back. I felt served and summoned. I was the chosen one to fulfill the deed. The obligation of my mother's concerns was deposited on my lap, into my account with no approval or signature - a customary requirement, I thought.

There was no choice. I was the undocumented creative, living in a traditionalist world illegally. I had to be sacrificed for the good of the whole. The limo was the least dangerous place to wait before the authorities of my fate caught up with me.

Stop it, stop it, stop it, I screamed inside myself. Where are you going with all this thinking? This is not the time to go crazy.

I took several deep breaths and told myself everything was going to be fine. My mother was like a bull for God's sake. I seriously believed she was too damn stubborn to give in to any serious illness. Finished. I would think nothing more into an uncertain future.

A pile of colored paint specs was scattered on my lap - enough of a gathering to make me stop picking. I brushed the colors off my skirt and looked out the window past my reflection. Everything I was familiar with wasn't there. The snow covered it up.

My stare was stuck and blurred everything outside. I blinked hard to clear my eyes. But the reflection took me in and replayed my last visit like an old movie.

I closed my eyes and heard a whisper so soft I could barely hear the words - I'm here. When my eyes opened the window reflected a girl, looking like myself, walking into at my mother's house in the middle of the night.

"I'm here. Mom...I'm here..."

The girl in the window's reflection had just opened the front door and stood in an entry motionless. She had appeared overwhelmed by the commotion before her.

3.
A MONTH EARLIER

[Images crushed up against each other
like a mob of angry protestors carrying
all the obvious signs I neglected to see.
I was there just a month ago.]

Looking back from outside myself.
I am the girl...

"I'm here. Mom, where are you?"

Inside all the fixtures were working hard - everything was on its highest volume. Lights from all the shaded and florescent fixtures loudly went about their business of changing night into day bright.

The girl had slowly brushed the snow-wet hair out of her face and leg slammed the door behind her. The heat appeared to have suffocated her face at first - her eyes looked squeezed and sucked dry. Chimes from a standing old clock in the entry vibrated a nervous sound without the help of time telling it what to do. Loud sounds, busy in various conversations, over-talked each other from another room.

A radio voice had babbled about the snow, *"770 customers are still without power. A few isolated areas will be restored on Saturday late in the afternoon. It's a bad night to travel folks."* – The television's Ben Matlock just reported to the police, *"Lucy's dead. She died in her sleep sometime last night, in that beach house of hers in*

Texas." – The radio's traffic reporter talked over Ben... *"No fatalities. A semi-truck overturned on the Stevenson near the Pulaski exit."* TV Ben added *"Yup, dead. She has a husband living in Mexico. We need to find him."*

An old boombox was playing gypsy music in the background. Music played by Stephan.

Every inch of air transmitted some sound. The noises tripped over each other demanding the girl's hearing attention.

Stephan was the girl's uncle, a brilliantly intense musician who pounded on the piano like a prizefighter. He was an impressive classical pianist who performed in a number of Chicago clubs and gypsy bars in Chicago. He was expressively dramatic and perpetually on stage. Years ago, Stephan would take the girl to bars that had pianos. He coached her to ask the bartender if her uncle could play Happy Birthday for her on their piano. More than often, they said yes, except for once. "Didn't you have a birthday last week?" The girl was quick. "Oh no, that was my twin sister."

Stephan would start with playing Liszt's version of Happy Birthday that went on for hours. He dazzled his audience and won over their admiration as he changed their corner bar into Carnegie Hall. The paid musicians who were on a cigarette break would often get angry. When Stephan finished, he bowed profusely to standing ovations and requests to continue. He smiled modestly and left with the night's tips. He was a colorful character who brought music, volume and division among the family traditionalists.

The girl moved slowly into the entry hall. Her purse strap slid off her shoulder. She had brushed away the outside off her coat and had extended her hand to the wall for balance while she toe-pushed the UGGs off her feet.

Looking up at the landing's rail, the girl saw her mother, standing in a chenille robe and wearing a glorious pair of Valentino turquoise pumps. Her hair was pinned and pressed down in parts like a pancake. At the top of her head, a heavy blue hairnet delicately sat on its side, proper-like, adding a French foreign accent to her appearance. Under the robe, one could see that the girl's mother was completely dressed in church clothing and appeared fully prepared at a second's call to attend any event or service that she possibly forgot. But for now, a tied flowered apron kept everything she had together and gathered at the waist.

The mother rubbed the back of her hand on her apron leaving breadcrumb prints in its ruffles.

"I'm so glad you're here. I was worried. I said to Jesus to listen to me and bring my daughter home safely." Without taking a breath, she changed her tone and added, "Where's your driver? Where's Jaidee? I got some candy for him."

"He's... He's gone, mom."

The mother paid no attention to the girl's words and dangled a small plastic bag over the railing. The zip-lock was filled with silver wrapped candies, hard candies with chocolate mint inside. There were cases of these candies in the basement. The girl filled 142 bags with those candies during her previous visit.

"Go see if he left the driveway. He needs to turn around. Hurry, go catch him."

"Mom, he's gone already. It's snowing and freezing cold out there. He's not going to turn around anyway, even if he..."

The house was warm and sunny. The mother could only appreciate her own generosity at that moment. But even those concerns about the candy or the driver didn't stay long in her head.

"Are you hungry? I have the Jello you love with the baby oranges stuck inside." The girl loved that style of Jello... when she was five.

"Come, come. I'm in the middle of making my cabbage horns." Fingers with flour and breadcrumbs stuck to the tips, twirled themselves in the air with the mother's directional instructions. It was all in the wrist.

The girl followed her mother into the kitchen, a small corner section of a larger room. Her mother's walk and talk were synchronized and centered in her course. The cooped-up odors of onions, cabbage and olive oil lay around lazy-like in the air.

"I couldn't sleep. I kept on thinking about..." the mother stopped for a moment; her thought lost its way and sunk out of sight like colored glass chips in a kaleidoscope.

"Mom... Mom."

She just moved on, oblivious to her lost thought and to the girl.

Off to the side was an aisle kitchen area. A long counter sat under an uninterrupted line of windows.

Only two had the power to be opened. Old paint from old painters held the others shut.

On the counter was a radio with oversized knobs that moved its needle easily from station to station. It kept the mother company; kept her informed. The radio voice inside the black box would tell her the locations of all the backed-up traffic jams and accidents in Chicago. When she wasn't home, the voice would talk to prospective burglars outside the house and tell them not to come in.

The room was cooking-warm and disheveled. The girl looked for someplace to plop down her purse. The counter was cluttered with thick-rimmed bowls filled with half mixed ingredients from family recipes. Flour and powered sugar dusted the counter from one end to another. The crushed nuts, cabbage slivers and poppy seeds found themselves in each other's mix.

"The pharmacist lady at Walgreens, her name is Evelyn something... she's always so nice to me; well her husband is gonna die this week so I'm baking two trays of cookies for the wake; a plate of cabbage horns and some baby hamburgers. They can just pick up the foods with their fingers, easy-like, as not to interrupt their grieving."

"Mom... what are you talking about? Evelyn who? And how do you know her husband's going to die?'

The mother paid little attention to her questions but the girl continued asking.

"Is he sick? Do you know this pre-deceased person? Do you even know what he looks like?"

"No. I never met him personally, not face-to-face. I'll meet 'em at the wake. Questions, questions, questions - don't worry me with all your questions."

The mother turned her body to end the questioning and continued talking.

"It's gonna be a two-day wake for sure. I think he's an important man. Do you remember Emil's wake and his funeral?"

The mother was giddy. Her adrenaline was pumped. She loved funeral-talkin'.

The girl avoided getting into the conversation. She walked to the refrigerator and opened its door looking for something, perhaps answers, possibly some insight or a beer.

"Maybe you had already moved to California when he died. He had fifty-seven cars in his funeral procession - fifty-seven, mind you."

She got chills talking about such processional events. The number of cars in one's funeral procession affirmed the dead person's importance, his accomplishments, how much he or she was loved.

The mother moved closer to her daughter who was reaching far back into fridge's lower shelf and leaned over to get closer to the girl's ear.

"I hope when I die I have fifty-eight cars. You got to promise me there will be at least one car more than fifty-eight."

The girl looked at her mother somewhat relieved, "Now that's the mother I know. You want to out-car some poor dead guy!"

The mother turned herself back to the counter attempting to remember what she was doing.

"Your father only had seventeen... but he had a bad attitude. You can't expect many cars at your funeral when you got a bad attitude."

The girl pulled out a bottle of Saris beer and a juicy lemon.

"Mom, please shut off that damn radio. How can you even think when that radio is yakking all the time? Music would be one thing but traffic and more traffic and more traffic and then the pile-ups and..."

The mother wiped the radio clean of any settling flours and lowered its volume a tiny bit. Then she carefully put away the recipe for her cabbage horns that was written in her mind.

"You have to come with me to the wake. You might meet someone."

"Seriously? I don't think so mom. Something about meeting a guy at a wake that gives me the chills… it all sounds so creepy."

"Well you aren't going to meet a nice man when you continuously hang around those artist people who don't have jobs or a pot to piss in – sitting in those coffee places with people who talk about all kinds of worldly things and new ideas that don't mount to nothin'. You think I don't know what goes on in those places. A lot of talkin' about useless stuff."

Violet rinsed her hands in warm water. White flour turned to paste and pealed off her skin into the sink's hole.

The girl appeared to be more comfortable and began moving around the room looking for an open space to sit.

In the corner a small round table with its partnering chairs was cluttered with papers, magazines and third-noticed bills. Next to the table was a couch where family dramas and secrets were stuffed under its upholstery, tiny pink and green flowers embroidered on satin fabric with wood trim that wrapped around the it's frame. Carved hand claws cupped the edges of the armrest.

In front of the couch was a short table. The table had a broken leg and looked lost in the room. It had a style that was all wrong and it wasn't just its obvious crippled leg. It was old and was originally in front of another couch belonging to the mother's sister who died years ago. Its formica wood was now too old and too tired to mimic real wood. The girl's father unevenly duct taped its broken leg back in place. Three matchbooks taped under the injured leg was part of the repair.

The couch and the table faced a boxy black working television sitting on top of a blond French provincial non-working counsel television. The counsel hadn't worked for years, but it was the youngest and least injured piece of furniture in the room. Violet bought this piece at the Merchandise Mart in Chicago. The girl remembered her mother standing and singing in front of the television to the national anthem that was played at the end of the broadcasting day. They stopped playing the anthem in 1974. The girl's mother just recently resurrected the patriotic practice. She would sing the anthem after the Matlock late night reruns.

"Mom, where's the remote?"

The girl's hand scanned under the couch pillows for the hard plastic box with the soft buttons.

"I'll get it. Wait a minute. Don't move anything." Violet had rushed nervously over to the couch.

"I'll get it. I'll get it. Move aside. Let me get it."

Under two pillows, under her purse, under wads of rolled Kleenex and tucked deep into the side's cushion, she had dug out the control.

"Why do you hide the remote?"

"People was stealing from me. I gotta be careful."

"But who would steal from you? You live alone...."

"Never you mind."

The girl didn't want to continue.

"You have to be more patient," she had told her daughter as she pointed the remote directly in the line of Ben Matlock and pressed on a button firmly. Ben talked louder. He had taken over the room shouting at his jury. The mother pushed more buttons, more firmly with a stern index finger. Finally, Matlock listened and lowered his volume.

"There. Is that better for you? This channel is for Ben MetLife. He's good."

She had put the remote in her apron pocket.

"Mom, it's Matlock. Ben Matlock... not MetLife."

[I replayed that night a million times over in my head, carefully watching that girl with her mother. Did I miss something?]

4.
DON'T LEAVE ME HERE

Weeee-oooooh! weeeee-oooooh! Blasting sirens and flashing lights cut through my window's reflection and raided everything; the girl and her mother, the floured counter and the room with the couch, all gone. I was left inside a warm limo staring at a cold window with no reflected memory.

The inside moisture slid everything down into the window's pocket. I shook my head from side to side, a kinder way of slapping myself silly into the moment in front of me.

Jaidee talked backwards to me in the mirror.

"An accident ahead Miz Suzka..." then slowly merged the moment into one lane with the other vehicles.

When we got closer to the accident the traffic tightened its grip. Lights flurried around a pile of trucks and cars coiled together. The merciful snow tried to cover their brokenness. A few people stood outside shivering. One man, younger, looked like a madman, his eyes in two black holes, yelling loudly with his hands. Another, a man in uniform pulled a woman out of a car. A policeman walked in front of our limo and extended his hand out signaling us to stop.

The cars, the trucks, the ambulances and the lights spread and stretched out like a canvas covering one side of the limo's windows. On the other side, the side where I sat, behind the glass a semi-truck pressed against all four windows. Everything once white disappeared. The sky was empty. All I could see were massive tires packed with chunks of snow frozen stuck in its wheels. Wheels that could run me over if they had a mind to, dragging my heart and my bloody guts to the city's vultures to dine on; if they had a mind to.

The snow turned to rain and came down like glass beaded curtains falling across the road. It clattered against the limo making a sound like sea pearls falling from the sky.

The policeman loudly waved at Jaidee.

"We are moving again Miz Suzka. Soon you will be to your maw'ter's home."

A small voice whispered inside me: *"I'm here..."*

*

From the street half the house looked abandoned. Window blinds were shut keeping the inside trapped. The house was bundled in snow. Heavy mounds sat on rooftop looking like visiting sea lions that stopped to take a rest before they returned to the ocean. The driveway was packed with snow and ice causing the limo to slide closer to the front door before its stop. The limo settled close to the front door.

"Jaidee, you don't have to help me with my luggage. It's too cold. Stay inside. I want to just slip out by myself."

"But Miz Suzka, don't you want me to take your baggages inside your maw'ter's home?'"

"No. Not this time. Thank you though. You are such a sweetheart. Besides, I am wearing warmer clothing than you. Just flip the trunk open. I'll get it myself."

Jaidee did not argue. He was never properly stubborn with me.

Jaidee twisted his torso and rested his full arm over his seat. I handed him his fare.

"Don't forget Miz Suzka, call me when you need to get back to dee airport. Or if you need a ride into the ceetee."

"I will. You know I always do."

"Tell your maw'ter 'Hello' and give her a big hug for me."

I didn't tell Jaidee my mother was not in the house. I didn't tell him about the accident, the fall. He would have worried.

Jaidee smiled and gave me that wink - the wink that always brought me back into the soul of the moment where everything was simple and clear.

The limo drove away. I held on to its red backlights until they turned into tiny wet crystals dissolving into the white. The snow wet my face.

I was in two minds. I desperately wanted to chase after him but I couldn't move, forward or back. I stood on the edge of decisions and looked around. The snow blurred what was ahead.

I hadn't a key to get into the house but remembered. *Yes, yes the door*, I forgot. Was that last week or was it two weeks ago. The break-in.

[She called me weeks ago
about the break-in. It was
early in the morning. My mother
never fully understood
the rules of the creatives...
Never call before noon.]

"Suzka, are you up... this is your mother calling. The front door is in pieces because of an axe broke it down. Get back to calling me. My number is 555-312-6013. This is your mother. Don't forget. Call me... 555-312-6013." Click.

The sound was loud and screechy in my dream. It had sliced though the air on a flock of razors. It was early, damn early even for a dream. The sound was of a woman whose voice had slaughtered all respectable dreams, leaving them dismembered – dreams looking for their endings in places where dead people might go to get some peace and quiet.

I was toasty warm under the stack of worn blankets and spotted cushioned pads used by movers for packing. Anything sticky and wet on top was paint from the night's incorrigible colors that hadn't enough time or patience to dry themselves.

Just the top of my head, above my nose was exposed to the elements.

I cracked open my eyelids and looked up cross-eyed at my bangs blowing in the breeze. It was morning and cold, cold for California. A breeze came from the open sides of a large roll-up door about ten feet away from my bed.

The roll-up was the main entrance into the studio, a rather large cement block structure with only one small window. The outside read Suzka Studio, white scribbled letters painted on a vertical black plank.

Under the covers, my ghostly friends to the likenesses of Picasso, Giacometti, Rauchenberg, deKooning and Gulley Jimson rolled over when they too heard my mother's voice.

The warehouse was wide and filled with color, barely a smidgen of the cinder walls poked through. Canvases stretched on their frames, still not quite ready to finish what they wanted to say, were piled everywhere. There were carpet tubes, sculptures, easels and coffee cups with paint stuck to its ears, tucked about the room. Everything was in the process of becoming something wonderful. I was part of the room; part of these runaway masterpieces, undisciplined, refusing to be captured and stretched.

"Suzka, this is your mother. Where are you? This is an urgency message. Call me right away. My number is 555-312-6013." Click.

There was no way in hell I was going to move any part of my body. The breeze, the cold and no coffee were solid reasons to stay buried. I scooted down deeper into my warm abyss and covered my head. For oxygen, I funneled a small opening big enough to let in just enough air to keep me alive. All outside sounds were muffled, as if a hand from behind the voice covered its mouth.

"Suzka, did you get my message I left on your phone to you? I'm going to church but I'll wait for you to call me before I'm leaving. This is your mother. My number is 555-312-6013." Click.

The words sat in the air waiting, looking around for someone to acknowledge its presence before the room had no choice but to absorb its' lingering sound.

"Suzka wake up. I forgot to telling you that five policemen were in my bedroom. They're all now gone. I was barely dressed and very close to naked. Call me as soon as you get this tape. My number is 555-312-6013. This is your mother. Call me." Click.

Oh God, two words that should never be in the same sentence, 'mother' and 'naked'.

My sleep shook me to wake. I got up, went to the bathroom and returned somewhere to my dreams unnoticed. At least I thought I did.

5.
THE BREAK-IN

[Based on police records, my mother's version and the artistic additions in color...the following five pages pertains to the actual break-in.]

"Mrs. Violet are you ok? This is the police."

The words got bigger as uniformed men walked through the house.

"Mrs. Violet, where are you?"

A voice turned the corner and walked towards Violet's bathroom.

The bathroom was poorly lit, cluttered and dated. Two of the six round bulbs refused to light. The counter was filled with beauty products: a sticky collection of dust-powered bottles with worn-off expiration dates. The jars of cream and moisturizers were kept close to Violet's reach. In the corner a heavy crystal vase held stemmed old hairbrushes with smashed down bristles. Next to the vase was an old cigar box of lipsticks dating back to the sixties. Most of them held only a smidgen of lip color and were deeply dimpled into their metal holders. Scattered within the clutter were three, possibly four green bottles of Campho-Phenique. Violet believed the C-P healed all bruises and cuts and healed earaches, leg cramps, broken bones, migraines, polio and gunshot wounds.

On occasion, I had been a witness to my mother's morning ritual. I moved 2000 miles away years ago but the process had never changed. She would start with the lotions and move to the moisturizers and then to the beige creams. After she more than adequately covered every facial corner, she would reach for the lipstick and blot a series of small dabs, three exactly on each creamed cheek that she would then smear up into her cheek bones, high into the illusion. Then slowly and as soft as a whisper she removed a tattered nylon hair net that covered her head. During the sleep, the net protected some parts of her upsweep-style and smashed down other parts. With a ballpoint pen she always kept on the counter, she lifted the flat sections and patted down other parts in order to even-out her style. Her hands moved fast with direction and purpose, moving in and out. In her time, everything would come to an abrupt calm. She glanced sideways out of her eyes at the mirror accessing the reflection of her work. For the grand finale, she spat twice into her fingers and rolled the spittle juice around evenly. When the tips were adequately lubricated, she gathered a cluster of stubborn hairs from each side of her forehead and twisted them inward into a curl on each side like quotation marks. Her spit kept them in place.

The final application, her signature, placed a smidgen of Campho-Phenique behind each ear as if it were Macy's perfume. Everyone knew when Violet was near. There was a stringent medical aroma that had stuck around long after she left the room. The vapors had stuck to the walls and to my nasal passages for years. To this day, when I think of my *morning-mother*, the hairs in my nose quiver.

*

"Mrs. Violet?"

A tall figure, a heavenly vision backlit in shimmering white filled the bathroom door's frame. Violet was startled and silent. She read of such visions but never thought... Violet dropped out of her body like a little doll. Looking up, her mouth opened but it was empty. In the supple light there flashed an image of Saint Michael.

Violet was much shorter than her sainted visitor. If she wanted to, if she could, if the angels would help her, she would let him hold her close, allowing his saintly chin to rest virtuously on her head.

The silhouette moved closer into his body. His head blessed with glassy black curls, his face was clean of hair and angled. He was pressed and ironed and carried a sword leathered at his waist. He wore the uniform of the city, a shiny dark gabardine. A metal flash of light came from his chest that made Violet blink. The metal was gold and reflected his number, 434.

"Mrs. Violet, are you ok?" He repeated the question.

The strange voice slapped everything holy out of Violet. The angels flapped their silken wings and flew away taking with them all thoughts of Saint Michael.

"Oh yes. Yes. I'm ok."

Violet backed up a bit and clutched her bathrobe's collar against her chest making it impossible for her breasts to see what was going on. Meanwhile, the fumes from the Aqua Net hairspray and her C-P perfume were fighting for air rights.

"Violet, the girls at Life Alert have been calling you on your speaker box but you hadn't answered. They called our police department to check on you. We rang the doorbell and knocked a number of times. We had no choice but to break in. We're glad to see you're not hurt."

Getting into the house could not have been an easy task. The *wood-n-chain* concoction prevented anyone on the outside from opening the door; a heavy metal chain looped several times around the doorknobs and a two-by-four butted between the door and a stair railing six feet away.

"Oh my God, I didn't hear a thing."

The policeman removed the cap from his head and rubbed the hard red line it sliced into his forehead. He smiled widely; his white teeth filled his face, his skin was golden dark

"You had everyone pretty worried. When we received no response, we had no choice but to break in."

For some reason, he needed to repeat the break-in part. Perhaps she didn't hear it the first time.

"Unfortunately, your door is in pieces."

Violet covered herself and tightened her robe.

"Come, come... let's go into the kitchen, I will make you something to eat."

"We can't Miss Violet, we have a full day of work ahead of us."

Saint Michael put his policeman's cap back on his head and moved aside making room for this tiny woman to pass. Four thick policemen in heavy uniforms and leathered pouched guns stood just outside her room waiting for direction.

"Oh my dear. There are so many of you. And you all came to rescue me. Come. Follow me." She waved her hand in the air and moved into action.

They fell like dominoes into her easiness as she passed by swinging her arms and talking.

"I have cream puffs in the freezer. But if you don't have time, let me at least give you some bags of candy?"

Violet turns and looks up at Michael.

"You count them. I want to make sure they all get a

bag. Are any of you policemen diabetic? I have sugarless."

[The image of the St. Michael's visit
wore off the next day but the notion
of the door's reckless destruction,
stuck with my mother for months.
Duck-tape covered the evidence.

*

My body pushed on the door that easily released its duct-taped closure.

The house was empty of real life but warm. The sounds and lights were working hard as if someone was there. A flickering glow from the television filled the ceiling. I walked up the dark stairs and moved toward the kitchen. Muffled conversations from the TV and radio didn't stop talking at my arrival. They have been warning prospective burglars not to come into the house since Violet left to go to church two days ago.

It was too early to go to the hospital. It was still the tail-wagging end of yesterday. My phone said 4:40am. The fresh white snow looking through the windows dimly lit the counter and created a suitable amount of light for moving around. A clipped-closed bag of pretzels was stuffed in the corner. I love pretzels. In one rhythmic sweep, I turned off the radio, snapped up the bag and grabbed a beer out of the fridge.

Exhausted but not quite ready to officially collapse into sleep, I plopped down on the sofa, covered myself with a blanket and turned my head toward the TV. Matlock was on.

*

I slept deeply on the sofa until my body shook me into waking. The jolt rattled all dreams out of my head. In my hand the remote control was stuck. Matlock left the box hours ago. I rolled on the sofa to face its back and hide from the morning. Its tiny pink flowers and green leaves lay flat on my eyes wallpapering my sight. The smell of paint, the weight of my splotched blankets, the cinder-block darkness was missing.

The room was yellow bright. The night found a few places to hide but for the most part, it was packing up ready to leave soon. California suns were never quite as rude. The sun out west would wait outside until I cranked up the roll-up door and allowed their light to start my day.

I slid my feet onto the floor, sat up and looked around. It was loudly quiet, a silence that screamed and pulled at my hair. Half my face felt dented, filled with bed wrinkles, my eyes were glazed. I put my hand to the top of my head for reassurance - a deflated bungeed mass of blond-red-black hair fountained loosely, sliding off the side of my head. I could have easily been compared to the portraits painted by Georg Baselitz or Francis Bacon, which I found awkwardly interesting.

The sun and its overbearing brightness took over the room. I released the latch for a window blind closest to me, which made it slam down hard onto the windowsill.

Where were my sunglasses? Questions were wrinkled in yesterday.

The morning waited for the coffee to stop perking before it would explain everything to me.

I showered, brushed and peed; then, dressed, layered and sunglass'd myself in record time, a practiced accomplishment. The morning's mission came in sight as I skipped down the steps, claw-clipping my hair to an upsweep ponytail.

At the stairs' landing, I got a pull from under my feet that knocked me over. The bottoms of my boots got stuck in its steps. My body flipped forward, bounced, then tumbled and eventually hit the floor hard.

I was ambushed. As if I was attacked by a pod of extremely strong and sticky octopi. The more I moved the more their tentacles tightened their grip, sucking and pulling me down. I was lying in a pile of duct-tape, tape that had ripped away from the door, the same door I pushed open to get into the house the night before.

"Fuckin' Duct Tape. Fuckin' stupid tape…

I tried to rip off the trappings but it only tightened its grip. My hands turned and twisted, my legs were stuck in place.

"...and what in the hell kind of protection is this? Any maniac in the middle of the frickin' night, could have broken-in easily and rob me. They could have knocked me out cold, tied my hands and feet with all this frickin' duct tape... and ransacked the house."

My body contorted like a gymnast. Strips of the tape fixed itself to my hair and hung loosely down my shoulders looking for more of me to capture. With all my force I crunched some of the tape into a ball as if I were fighting for my life and slap-slammed other pieces back onto the door.

"Horrible hellacious people could have slit my throat, ripped off my cloths, ravaged my body and left me for dead... blood everywhere. ...I hate this fuckin' tape. I swear I hate this frickin' fuckin' tape."

After my release, I rubbed the bumped parts my head to prevent any bruising and continued walking down the side steps toward the basement door to exit. Outside my mother's car sat under a pile of snow.

[The church ladies previously drove the car to the house. No butt, other than my father's (occasionally) sat in the driver's seat before that day.]

6.
A BOTTICELLI MOMENT

Patient Room #404: "Tay took your mother dow'na-stairs for somma tests." The voice came from a bed closest to the door.

The occupant of the bed was a perky woman who appeared to be good at camouflaging her health. She raised her blanket and repositioned its landing over her legs, then ran her hands over the creases to smooth out the surface. A curtain separated the two beds for cottoned privacy.

"Dow'na-stairs... Tay took her toda elevator and lowered her to doz blood suckers on ta ground level."

She confidently snickered to herself, amused at her own comic sense of humor.

The lady of the voice looked at me with all her eyes and ears. Obviously, this was a versed woman who had accumulated a number of hospital experiences. She was a bit older, in her seventies, the very late seventies perhaps. Her hair was short, curly, salt and pepper in color, more salt than pepper. Her cheeks were her most prominent feature. Round and puffy, stuffed with outspoken jabberwocky nonsense as well as tiny bits of wisdom stuck far back around her molars. With absolutely no control on her part, her words fell out randomly whenever she opened her mouth

"My name is a Josephine." The little lady looked up, raised her brows and opened her eyes wide.

"Gull bladder." Spoken as if they were her rank and serial number.

Josephine went back to folding and shook her head. She pushed out her lips and melodically slipped in a diagnostic opinion.

"She deaden' look very happy."

"What... what did you say? Your name is Josephine? Hello Josephine, I'm... How did you know she was my mother?"

"Honey, I knowz those things."

"That's nice. Well... where did you say they took my mother?"

"Dow'na-stairs. Ask one of ta nurses outside to give you directions, but make sure they don't point you toda wrong elevator."

Josephine waved her finger in the air adding credibility and weight to her words.

"You canna get lost in dis place if you take ta wrong elevator. One of doz elevators canna take youz directly toda morgue - not ta any stops."

As Josephine nodded her head and fiddled with the top hem of her blanket creating a neat fold-over edge, she added under her breath,

"They donna tell anybody dat. You just end up dare. The morgue. And ya don't want to go dare."

"Thanks... Josephine, and thanks for the information."

“Shez be ok honey. While youz out dare, tell the nurz I need my medzine.”

*

The elevator's sliding doors opened into a long corridor. The light was strikingly different, dim. All the sounds whispered. Directly in front of me was a line of cushioned chairs filled with people dressed in partially opened hospital gowns - some wore bandages and surgical masks, others coughed, snored in wheelchairs or read old magazines with torn out pages. All of them had paper wristbands.

At the far end were double doors with head sized windows for viewing. A hand- sanitizing dispenser was respectfully walled next to the doors. I pushed on the dispenser's tail and spread the goop of white foam around my hands and then elbowed the two doors open.

The room inside was large and fluorescent bright with long metal tables in sheeted cubicles that corralled the room. Doctors in scrubs and white coats rushed through the area. Nurses hovered over patients, some stood by monitors, others tap-slapped wrists to wake up sleeping veins.

I looked around. My head followed the moaning sounds and voices from behind the curtained cubicles.

"Is anyone out there who could help me? Could someone please help me." ...while another screamed "Jackasses. They're all a bunch of jackasses!"

Groaning and whimpering, intercoms paging doctors, static noises from police radios stuffed my head. Buzzing alarms went off telling the nurses that transparent bags filled with medication were done. Pop, fizz from a soda can being opened came from around the corner where an older man sat slouched in a chair next to his bandaged wife. They shared a lemon soda.

In the center of the room computers, monitors and files were lined on counter tops and manned by the commanding nurses - nurses who ordered the airborne illnesses and contagious diseases to stay in their curtained cubicles. Everything was recorded.

I stopped the first blue, cotton-starched young man that walked passed me.

"I'm looking for my mother... Violet... a sweet little old lady about this high."

The orderly looked at me. He didn't have to say a word. Thoughts running in his head exposed themselves like a flasher at a train station. His body told me, *No one with that description or sweet disposition is here but there is a 'Violet' in cubicle four.*

The nice young orderly said nothing. His face did all the talking. He pointed to one of the curtained cubicles on the opposite side of the room.

I dragged my body past the nurses' station and stopped in front of the only cubical on that side of the room. The smell of antiseptic and hygiene products irritated my nose. Slowly I parted the cubicle's curtain and slid my head inside.

"Oh my God."

The woman in front of me was stark naked, sitting on a metal table covered partially with butcher-like paper, clutching a black purse under her breasts.

"Oh my God.... what in the hell...?"

I scooted my entire body further into the cubical and made sure the curtain was closed behind me.

"Mom… what ... "

I could barely talk.

"Where in the hell are your clothes? Didn't they give you something to wear? They must have given you a hospital gown."

My mother sat straight, proper-like but bare-assed and suctioned to the un-papered part of the table. Her leather purse was sweat-stuck to her belly; her knuckles were white from gripping its straps. The purse was the last thing she would let anyone take from her. The purse covered her tabernacle'd privates.

"Suzka, thank God and all the crazy saints you're here."

My mother raised the volume of her voice high enough for the entire ER to hear.

"These jackasses took my clothes. I want my clothes! I want to go home! Nobody will listen to me!"

She caught her breath and lowered her volume.

"Find my blue blouse; the one with the pearl buttons and my black skirt (pause) and my girdle. Find my girdle. They stole my girdle. I bet they stole my girdle. Jackasses."

Her hands were tempted to raise themselves in protest but her purse straps and religious fervor wouldn't let them go.

I was dumbfounded.

The image of my mother naked stuck in my eyes and had no intention on moving. I should have been upset, but at who? ...my mother? the doctors? myself? I waited outside my head for a reaction, a sensible reaction. But my only thought was... how pretty my mother looked, how extraordinary beautiful.

The woman in front of me, inside my mother's skin looked as if she were the long lost queen of the seas – an image not like an illustration in a magazine but more like a Botticelli painting, 'The Birth of Venus'.

[Botticelli's Birth of Venus is one of the most treasured artworks of the Renaissance. In it the goddess Venus, known as Aphrodite emerges from the sea upon a shell aligned with the myth that explains her birth. Her shell is pushed to the shore from winds being produced by the wind-gods in amongst a shower of roses. As Venus is about to step onto the shore, a Nymph reaches out to cover her with a cloak.]

"Why are you looking like that? Snap out of it. I need you to find my clothes."

I wanted to get to a doctor but I couldn't get myself to leave. There was this disheveled, almost distorted beauty about my mother. She dove again into more airy chatter that I heard at a distance. I stood there leaning back against the current, watching the waters where the Venus in my mother sat.

"And what are you wearing? Is that paint on your skirt? Don't you have any clean clothes? I didn't raise you like this. I always made sure you and your sisters had clean nice cloths. You girls were so cute."

She went away, somewhere for a bit. I dare ask.

"Where's that cute pleated skirt I got you for Christmas?" It was at the Salvation Army; a routine drop my little sister and I had made after every gifted holiday.

"Mom this skirt is perfectly clean. It just has a little paint on it."

"Oh forget it for now. Let's just get out of here. My clothes must be somewhere. Hurry. You're here now. Go… go tell them we're going home."

"Mom, calm down. You're here for good reason. You're here because you fell. Do you remember that you fell?"

I removed the Botticelli and Venus images from my eyes and paid closer attention to my mother's bruises. The skin around her right eye was black and purple. Her iris was moist and blood red. A large bandage covered a large bulge on her forehead. A few blood spots made their way through the gauze. She looked like she'd been mugged. The bruise made me lightheaded.

"What fall? All I know is somebody stole my clothes." Screaming louder and more agitated, she continued. "and they won't give them back to me."

Violet lowered her voice and directed her attention back to me. "Where is my... ah... you know the... ah... what you do… um, you know the thing that moves you around... You know what I mean? The thing. The thing that you get into..."

"Your car?"

I guessed.

"Yes the car. What ya think I was talking about. Do ya think I was NOT talking about the car?"

I never ever saw my mother this confused, this disoriented.

"Mom. You have to wait here a bit. A doctor should come by pretty soon and he'll tell us what's going on."

I collected my thoughts and returned to my mother's nakedness...

"Let me find you a blanket."

"Go. Go. Go… and ask them to turn up the heat. Its damn cold in here."

I moved a small part of the curtain a tiny bit to the side and peeked my head out into the room. The lights were burning bright. I wanted to vomit. My head tunneled my vision and focused my thought. Blanket. Blanket. Find a blanket.

A few feet away were a stack of sheets lying on the nurses' counter. Good enough. I grabbed one and turned back quickly, Venus returned to my mother's face.

"Here mom, let's put this sheet around you until we find your clothes. How do you feel? This bruise looks bad. Does it hurt? It doesn't look good mom. Are you sure you're ok?"

"Of course I'm ok."

Violet never let herself get sick. She always stayed enormously healthy popping discounted vitamins and following the advice from cutout articles found in her Natural Health magazines. Campho-Phenique, vinegar, cola syrup and onion peelings took care of nearly all the semi-serious illnesses.

Violet looked around the cubical agitated.

"This place is filled with jackasses!"

A nurse walked in, a doctor followed. He pulled the curtain back behind him covering Violet's partially naked breasts from the rest of the room.

"Hello Violet. How are you feeling?"

"Just fine." she answered in a fake full-dressed voice. Violet sat up straight and looked at the white-cloaked man directly in his eyes.

"We are ready to go. My daughter is here to take me home."

"Well, Mrs. Violet, you're pretty sick. We're going to keep you here for a few more days."

"Listen Doctor, my daughter is standing right there. See that girl?" She released one finger that gripped the straps of her purse and pointed it at me.

"That's my daughter. She flew here all the way from California and she's gonna take care of me to my home. Now if you can find my clothes, I'd be grateful then I can get out of here."

Violet moved her attention toward me. "Give him some of those candies and let's go home."

"Are you Violet's daughter?"

"Yes."

"Your mom is very sick. We ran a number of tests and did a spinal tap, which is why she is so irritated... and naked. We gave her a gown. The nurses helped her put it on but I am not sure what happened to it. I'll ask the nurse to bring in another gown."

The doctor continued in more seriousness.

"Your mother has meningitis-encephalitis."

I felt the heavy weight of those words without really knowing what was behind them.

"It is the inflammatory disease of the membranes that surround the brain as well as the spinal cord. In your mother's case, she probably had the infection for months. The infection has caused a rapid onset of dementia."

I couldn't find any words. I dropped my head and studied my mother over my eyeglasses. There was no sign of a question in her eyes.

The doctor said, "We'll keep her here for now."

His words felt like hands that covered my ears. He kept talking... it didn't seem to make any difference. My ears stopped all words coming through its canal.

"Has she traveled abroad in the last six months? Has she been around anyone who's been sick, has herpes, anyone with the mumps, or HIV?"

Oh my god... where is this going? Does this woman in front of him look like she's a world traveler? Does she look like she would go to some foreign drug infested country on vacation? Does she look like a smuggler, a mule? For Christ sake, what in the hell is he talking about?

Images flashed quickly of my mother sharing needles with other church ladies after mass. You never really know a person.

"Has she been outside near water, near mosquitoes?"

"The fourth of July picnic." The half naked woman spoke.

Violet participated in the conversation only when it had some pleasant interest to her.

"We had over seventy-five people come to our Fourth of July family reunion. Tell him Suzka. It was the biggest crowd we ever had. Some people came from as far as Texas."

She turned her full attention toward me for some sort of clarification. "Remember Suzka? Tell him. There were seventy-five... tell him there were seventy-five."

The doctor added, "She must have had this virus for months. She appears to be showing signs of being in the moderate stages of dementia. But unfortunately with this virus you will soon see a quick progression in both her memory loss and communication. We can treat the meningitis-encephalitis but there is nothing we can do for the dementia. Does she live alone?"

"Yes." My response was slow, the 'yyye...' extended in the air as if it were standing on a bridge's ledge; the remaining 'sss' jumped to its death.

"Do you live near your mother?"

"No. I... I live in California."

"Well, she cannot live alone anymore."

The words *'she cannot live alone'* piled up on top of each other and stuck in my head. I could not breathe. I felt faint and damp. I blinked fast as not to cry.

"For now we'll start her on antibiotics that we will give to her through an IV for about ten days. This procedure we can start today in the hospital."

Meningitis is an inflammation of the membranes (called meninges) that surround the brain and spinal cord and is caused by bacterial or viral infections.

Encephalitis is inflammation of the brain. The leading cause of severe encephalitis is the herpes simplex virus. Other causes include enterovirus infections or mosquito-borne viruses. The diagnosis is usually made by performing a lumbar puncture (spinal tap). Encephalitis with meningitis is known as meningoencephalitis. This viral infection that affects the central nervous system can cause rapidly progressive dementia.

Dementia is not a specific disease. It's an overall term that describes a wide range of symptoms associated with the decline in memory or other thinking skills severe enough to reduce a person's ability to perform everyday activities.

People with dementia may have problems with short-term memory, keeping track of a purse or wallet, paying bills, planning and preparing meals, remembering appointments or traveling out of the neighborhood. While symptoms of dementia can vary greatly, at least two of the following core mental functions must be significantly impaired to be considered dementia: memory, communication and language, ability to focus and pay attention, reasoning and judgment and visual perception.

Many dementias are progressive, meaning symptoms start out slowly and gradually get worse.

Alzheimer's disease accounts for 50 to 70 percent of cases. Other common types include vascular dementia (25%), which occurs after a stroke, Lewy body dementia (15%), which refers to both Parkinson's disease dementia and dementia with Lewy bodies - abnormal protein deposits that disrupt the brain's normal functioning changes the way muscles work.

Violet's dementia was caused from Meningitis-
Encephalitis.

[That summer, before my mother's illness
two things happened: Hurricane Katrina hit the
Gulf Coast causing severe damage and Harry Potter
returned to Hogwarts fighting dragons.

"If your name is chosen, there is no turning back.
As from this moment, the Triwizard Tournament
has begun." - Albus Dumbledore]

7.
THE TRANSFER

A nurse led me to a small room about the size of a broom closet. The space was barren and beige with no windows and only one framed print on the wall of what looked like the Niagara Falls. It was god-awful ugly, flat, no life, no passion. I know for sure Picasso and Gulley Jimson would have hated it.

Under the 'Falls' was a table longer in its length than its width. Two chairs sat on opposite side at the table's length.

"There will be someone here shortly to help you with your mother's transfer."

Transfer? What is she talking about?

Before I got a chance to put my words together the door closed any opening for questions and the walls sealed themselves around me. Did she say transfer? Something instinctively made me stare up to the ceiling's corners expecting to find one of those tiny cameras they use in interrogating rooms at police stations.

In a short amount a time, the hospital's discharge nurse walked into the room and closed the door behind her - a slim young lady in her late twenties with pointy cone breasts. She was very pretty but if you needed to identify her to the authorities as a missing person, her breasts would be her most distinguishing feature, in addition to a scribbled tattoo on her neck that slid under her cardigan.

She smiled at me modestly - a cute little smile, just enough to uncover the tip of one tooth.

She brought in with her a clipboard and laid it on the table in front of me. Its metal gums bit down on a number of hospital forms and notepapers.

"Hello, my name is Lucy."

"Hello." The word came out of my mouth like a prisoner walking to his execution.

"We started your mother on intravenous antibiotics in the ER but we are unable to keep her here at the hospital for the full ten day treatment. We need to move her to another facility, probably by the end of this day. Right now we're checking with all our affiliate rehabilitation centers. When a bed is available, we will transfer her by ambulance."

"Move her... why can't she stay here?"

"She really doesn't need the full hospital care and your insurance would never cover it."

"But she's sick. Very sick from what the ER doctor told me. Go ask him. Really."

"I can assure you the rehab center we are waiting to hear from is well-equipped to care for your mother.

I hate when they shorten serious words - 'rehab' for rehabilitation as if it's a playful nickname, and in this case 'rehabilitation center' meant nursing home. This was bad. This was going to be very bad.

"But... " I felt the bones of her tiny hand reach across the table and pat my arm.

"Everything will be fine. They will continue the series of IV medications for ten days and then you can take your mother home. This gives you enough time to prepare for her return."

Her hand returned to the clipboard. Her eyes looked down into her readers.

"It is written here that you will be staying with your mother and that you will also be hiring an additional care giver to help you. Is that correct?"

"Well..." She could have been speaking Swahili.

"You fully understand that your mother will need around the clock care, don't you?"

A pause.

"You will need help."

A longer pause.

"You will not be able to take care of her by yourself." The slim young bearer of bad news waited for some response.

I opened my mouth but nothing came out. I didn't really listen to what she was saying but somehow I soaked it all up - the look, the tone in her voice, the smell air makes when it scrubs itself clean and the buzzing sound of the fluorescent lights. I was like a sponge. If anyone dared to squeeze me, everything would squish out and I would be just a puddle on the floor.

"Your mother's ten day stay at the rehab will give you enough time to get everything in order. But first we need to take care of the hospital's discharge paperwork and go over a few things."

There was a weighted knock at the door. In the crack of its' opening a head popped through. I was saved from continuing.

"Oh how wonderful. You came just in time. Suzka, this is Miss Blanchard. She works at the Aged Oaks Pavilion, the rehab center affiliated with our hospital. She's here with good news I hope."

Miss Blanchard shook my hand. Her fingers were like fat sausages and sweaty.

"Hello my dear... Suzka? Your name is Suzka?"

"Yes."

"What an interesting name. Is that Russian?"

"Thank you and no, it's Slovakian."

I could have said Chinese and her reaction would have been the same. She moved her attention and words toward Lucy.

"Yes, I have very good news and I brought all the paperwork with me to get things moving quickly."

Miss Blanchard was a stout, handsome woman with maroon hair pinned up in a pompadour hairstyle that looked old, as if the hairs had not moved or changed their direction since she was a young girl. She carried herself as the official ambassador for the Aged Oaks and smelled of a mixture of Jean Nate bath splash and Lysol disinfectant.

Lucy went out of the room to get another chair.

"I am so sorry to hear about your mother's illness."

She lifted her hands and held them close to her breast with the tips of her fingers pressed together as if they were in prayer.

"You need not worry. We have a bed available and we will be able to transfer your mother this afternoon. I can assure you that everyone at The Aged Oaks Pavilion will do everything they can to make her stay comfortable."

Lucy returned with a cushioned chair and placed it at the table's edge. Miss Blanchard kept on talking and sat down with no thought as to where her butt bottom would land.

"I brought the necessary papers with me for you to sign before we can admit your mother."

She made herself quite comfortable and pulled out a stack of papers from a folder with gold embossed lettering on its cover. In a matter of seconds the table was filled on both sides with notes, post-its and medical forms that I needed to read and sign.

"Tell me a little bit about your mother. You are her daughter right?"

"Yes."

"How lucky your mother is to have you. Is your father, Violet's husband, alive?"

"No. Not really." At this point, I didn't know what I was saying.

[Both ladies asked me a series of questions.
I felt absurdly close to tears. After what seemed like
hours of questioning, I broke. I squealed like a baby
and told them everything.]

8.
VIOLET'S STATS

My mother was the oldest of four children. Two girls came first and then two boys born twelve and thirteen years later. The first boy had been a difficult birth. According to my mother and my grandmother, a midwife had to use two gallons of lubricating oil. The boy baby, my uncle, the first son did not slide out like a pound cake from its pan, fresh out of the oven. The birth had left my grandmother ill with an un-reparable nervous condition that had never been actually diagnosed nor discussed. The older and wiser women in the neighborhood as well as the card-readers and fortunetellers told my grandmother that her suffering would be a *'cross she would have to bear'*. A year later, another brother came into the world without the oil. My mother somewhat raised her two brothers.

My mother's father was a strong prominent figure in his family and a Godfather to many extended Slovak families in Chicago's west side. He had found jobs and offered his home to many in trouble when times were hard. He was a statuesque man with a wide smile. I always believed he came from a long line of prominent gypsies in Europe. When I would ask about his people in Bratislava, my grandmother would tell me, "Hush now, don't talk such foolishness." and press one finger on her lips.

My grandmother didn't like gypsies. She believed they were thieves with slippery fingers. They were too wild, too filled with dance. Their glitter and gold she said would burn black holes in children's eyes. I believed my grandmother felt her husband put a spell on her that she could not break. All the saints in heaven could not protect her or break his power over her. She adored her husband, quietly.

The mystery, the gypsy colors of gold, the foolishness and his wide smile were the qualities I loved the most about my grandfather. Everyone loved him. After his death, Violet became the matriarch of the family.

In my mother's time, in Cicero, if a girl was not married by the age of seventeen, the family would enroll her in secretarial school to learn how to type and use a comptometer. They didn't go to art school, even if they were awarded a scholarship to the prestigious Chicago Art Institute. My mother loved art and loved to sketch. She learned how to use a comptometer and married at 22.

Violet had met her husband (my father) at a New Years Eve dance. He was a tall man, over six feet. His legs were long and smoothly covered the dance floor to any music played. He was light on his feet and could spin and turn-around any girl of any size and catch her in his arms. Violet, only five feet in her height would dance breathlessly with her handsome partner. Her feet barely touched the floor.

He had a chiseled face with deep-set eyes and perfect teeth. She called him Pavel. In six weeks, he would bring a box of candy to his 'soon to be' mother-in-law and solidify their engagement with the approval and blessing from his sweetheart's father.

It would be the first wedding for the Slovakian Godfather, a wedding for his first child, his oldest daughter. A wedding that would be celebrated in the grandest building in Cicero - The Hawthorn Pavilion.

The Pavilion was an old two-story frame building with two ballrooms. Each ballroom had an extraordinary large slick wood dance floor and a long open bar that extended the full width of the room. The carved mahogany bar was set back in an arched alcove. It was the largest building in Cicero that could accommodate huge family celebrations.

It had been an August wedding and it was hot, Chicago hot, Billie Holiday's '*Summertime*' hot. The air outside was thick. The sun had left slowly, exhausted from the humidity. Lazy fireflies had lowered the sky and talked a bit with the stars. The large windows in the Pavilion were as open as they could be, begging the outside air to come inside and dance with the music. Trees close by just watched - they had no rhythm.

There had been mountains of food, an unending flow of whisky and beer and loud music inside. The first floor had been decorated with white crepe paper streamers, strings of glass beads and tall vased calla lilies. At the far end of the room, a full band with cimbaloms, fujaras, violins and accordions played Slovak songs. Members from the band had taken turns singing garbled words into the microphone. Ladies in black dresses with sausage legs and disappearing husbands, sat on metal folding chairs near the band music, fanning themselves and singing only with the words they could remember.

Upstairs, another band played faster music for the younger crowd with English words. Their band played the latest Benny Goodman tunes with trumpets, clarinets, saxophones, and drums. The old ladies downstairs pointed to the jumpy ceiling above and whispered to each other, 'Swing' as if it was a dirty word.

On the main floor, set tables had circled around an open space, which created an area where the new bride and her husband danced the traditional first dance as a married couple. The other guests circled around and watched. Close family members waited only a short time before they would steal the dance away from the new couple. Uncles with deep affection for the bride would whisper in her ear their love and support "If he hits you, call me."

First and second generation aunts would in turn dance with the groom giving advice and simple threats.

"Be gentle and patient. I be over your house next week to find out if you listened well." The promised blessings were given to every bride and groom for generations.

Dancing went on for hours long into the night. Running children chased each other between the crowds. In the corner, a towering wedding cake nervously watched.

There was a steady stream of servers moving around the tables balancing heavy trays of food. Trays filled with bowls dripping in gravies on meats and sausages along with platters stacked with dumplings. On one side of the room was a line of tables filled with desserts made by family wives from handed down recipes - recipes they received from their husband's mothers that they will pass on to their children and to Violet.

Old men and uncles with soft legs that worked poorly leaned on the sticky bar, lifting shots of whiskey for luck, many babies and long lives. The many blessings given to the young couple, matching the promises made 'till death do they part'.

"Here's to Pavel and Violet. May they have many 'childrens' and health and happiness in their married lives together."

"Gratulujem"

"Nazdravie"

The many toasts spawned three girl babies.

[I went on and on with hardly a pause.
I gave the medical prosecutors everything they
had asked as if 'ratting out' on my mother
would end their questions.]

When the hospital ladies were done with me, I signed the papers that condemned my mother to a nursing home for the ten days and then left the room with remorse and guilt about everything I had ever done questionably wrong in my entire life. The walk toward the elevators was weighted by the deed. A strange quiet escorted my every step.

The hospital's bright white lights swept the floor soundlessly. Attendants prowled the halls opening doors sometimes and peering in. In the breath of its darkness you occasionally heard whimpering or soft sobs. Hospital corridors are strange places at night.

I couldn't swallow. My jaws clamped down tight. My head worked over the day. I couldn't believe what I heard but I had nothing else to confuse it with… *she cannot live alone.* The words fit a shape like a nut in a shell. Not too big but comfortably smug in its hallow cave.

Wait a minute I thought to myself. What does that really mean… *she cannot live alone?* What were the exact words? Maybe I wasn't listening carefully. Sometimes I do that. Sometimes my mind has a mind of its own. *I love that about myself.*

I didn't want to think about it much. It was too dangerous. It fixes it. It nails it down. But I found myself muttering with each step. *She cannot live alone… She cannot live alone?* Tears lost their way and filled my mouth. Someone inside said *don't you dare cry.*

I pushed the elevator button that arrowed down.

When the doors opened a man inside carrying a little girl in his arms moved slightly to the side. The little girl was tightly bundled in a pink padded jacket that went past her neck and hooded her head. A zipper and drawstring kept her stiff and fixed in place. The little girl stared at me, as did the balloon she was carrying by a string wrapped around her balled fist. Her stare continued for the longest time. Then, with no provocation on my part, she squished her lips together and pushed out her smart-ass tongue as far as it would go. I never had children myself but I believe pardoning parents would call that… 'she-missed-her-nap'.

The elevator hit the main floor with a jerk and opened its doors. I followed the sassy sack and her father out of the building.

*

It was a long day. Darkness was now complete. Great lumps of cold fell on top of me from under the night. There was nothing I could do to stop it nor did I want to. This was Chicago's cold, Chicago's snow.

There seemed to be a hint of magic to it all. In front of me were burning lights scattered all about the hospital's parking lot, all smiling down out of their glass eyes and casting a hard light on the covered tar. Their electric faces stood between me and the stars.

I vaguely remembered and at the same time, hardly recognized where I was. The parking lot was all white with scattered rectangle patches of blue-black where cars left to go home. Only a few mounds of white popped up from its flat landscape. One mound was in the shape of my mother's car.

I walked slowly to the covered sedan, brushed aside the snow parts hiding the driver side's door and slid inside. There I sat, in this cold metal containment, which seemed like hours waiting for the engine to clear its throat and blow in some warm air.

I bounced inside my skin and slapped my limbs together for friction warmth. The heater's control dial was on maximum heat as my breath vaporized the air and steamed the windows. The cold shivered my bones. I began to wonder how long it would take for bone marrow to freeze into tiny crystals. All I could do was wait, bounce and take tiny short breaths.

Thoughts of the day fell apart like a thousand snow crystals that went flying into the glass faces of the street lamps. The wipers helped and moved the snow away slowly at first and then nervously rushed it's sweep. I made them stop. Their nervousness irritated me.

I wanted to cry but it was too damn cold. Scared to death. My chest hurt. I felt like crying but wasn't sure. The cold air of the night blew into my head and made me dizzy. Those words took shape, like puppets and danced in my head – *'she cannot live alone... she cannot live alone.'* What was about to happen to me?

I felt shut off, squeezed and closed inside. I felt I was about to be compressed in a way that I wouldn't be able to do anything but think from the outside. My mentors, my ghostly friends, Picasso, Giacometti, Gully Jimson and DeKooning would sit in my brain like a lump of clay with nothing to say, giving no guidance. They would turn into thin paper passages bound in books, stacked on my bed 2000 miles away. I was alone.

My skin shivered. My heart beat like a toy that was wound too tight. My feet wanted to run, but where.

What was going to happen to me? Oh Jesus, why am I so Goddamn self-centered? ...another thing to worry about.

I felt like a corpse that spent a week in the bottom of an undisclosed river.

Shivering, I closed my eyes and used all my brains to go someplace other than where I was. Artists can do that if they had a mind to. I needed to transcend this cold, leave Chicago and run inside myself back to my studio where it was warm and foggy, with the sweet smell of paint drying and odors from dead fish carcasses squeezing their way through the sides of my roll up door.

transcend (trăn-sĕnd') *verb. transcend-ing*
– to go beyond the range or ordinary limits of something abstract, conceptual field, overpass; rise above (the universal or material existence)

9.
SUZKA AND THE CREATIVES

When I came out of my head, I was relieved. No doubt about it. I examined my diaphragm and felt a calming sensation, undoubtedly there was a physical sign of relief. I believed, as I walked into my virtual-studio that I had escaped a great deal of madness. I was finally home.

"Good lord where have you been. We ran out of wine." Oh my dear, dear Picasso.

Everything was just as it was that last night of painting. The paint cans were open, drooling their color. Brushes were either balancing themselves on the can's rim or bathing in one of the water buckets about the room.

"Suzka my dear, I have found myself to have been left in charge of the studio for the time of your absence and took full responsibility of your property."

"Of course Mr. Jimson, I would have not expected anything...." He cut my words short and continued.

"You needn't worry about your work. A good wall will paint itself. But upon further evaluation I... we have decided that your paintings need cacti and spiked grass, possibly some bald heads... and there needs to be dancing. Bosomy women dancing in bare feet. Yellow dark feet long with red nails."

Giacometti. "Ah yes, the imagination sustains creation and recalls it from the grave of memory."

Gulley Jimson pontificated, "Yes indeed. The angels must always be surprised when an artist dives head first into his paint and then with a twist of his imagination comes out again as bold as a eagle with wings bigger than the biggest in all the heavens."

Picasso's voice interrupted, "Suzka. Suzka... where is that girl? We need more wine, more Bordeaux, more imbibing spirits."

I had many mentors and colleagues. All are dead unfortunately. They lived with me and wasted no time in placing their opinions and theories about substance and creative worth inside my head.

"I like this," a comment from the other side of the room, Picasso pointed to a painting called the *African Skies*.

"Right here, you did not just paint a sun into a yellow spot..." overcome with his own theatrics, he paused and called on his hands to continue expressing his fervor. "...you transformed a yellow spot into a sun! Brilliant. I like very much."

Picasso then looked back at my *Adam and Eve* and moved closer into its space. His enthusiasm withered. Before I knew what was actually happening, he took my brush, wet with paint and in wide flying motions made bold color strokes across the canvas... without even asking.

At first I screamed but I could have fired a gun to his head and he wouldn't have heard a thing. Rain started and slapped the roof boorishly in support of my resentment. I cringed and tried to grab his arm. My anger tightened me, shut and closed me from anything outside my indignation. He kept yelling at me and at Adam and Eve, screaming in the air with his hands. "Blend them together, let Adam absorb Eve."

"Stop... you bastard! What are you doing? You've gone too far." Gulley Jimson badgered back. He had strong opinions about art.

Gulley was another close painter friend who lived in the pages of the literary world; he never got along much with other painters. He was quite melodramatic and forceful with his comments. Gulley admired, more than anything in the world, his own presence and particularly enjoyed the sound of his voice as he gushed over his armed opinions.

When the attack ended, Gulley moved his head toward my direction and with intrepid valor said... "My dear petsie, I will save your painting from this tyrant."

Picasso's hand brushed him off like a nasty fly hovering over a bowl of cheese balls.

"Go away. You cannot save something you don't understand."

"You make my guts wind." words Gulley used to point out not only his disgust toward Picasso but also to note his guts' distress at his opponent's bantering.

Picasso turned his attention and full body toward me as if we were already engaged in a long intimate conversation over a glass of Merlot. He lowered and spread out his words like soft butter on a croissant.

"Listen to me, my sweet goddess. You need to dissect all their parts and merge them in the garden, their Eden."

"Poppycock! And poppycock on your pissology and to your chopping women up into pieces like broken glass, scattering them into the trees."

Picasso boiled over like forgotten pasta left on the burner before it hit the sauce. He moved in on Gulley and poked him in the chest with his brush, my brush! Just inches away from his face, he pushed out his words. "You think too much and do so little!"

Gulley then grabbed a palette knife off my table and aimed it at Picasso's neck. "You arrogant son of a bitch. I'll carve out that manly apple from your bloody throat and feed it to the buzzards, you miserable chopper."

I thought I was going to explode. Everyone was talking and arguing in voices that resembled my own.

Pablo was furious and screamed back at Gulley.

"You're a foolish old man. Go back to your mural'ed giraffes and your circus models, your zebras and your mad drummers! AND what does it matter to you? It's not your painting. You seem to forget you're only a guest."

"I am no guest. I am Gulley Jimson... created by Joyce Cary... a literary genius, you blundering idiot. Suzka and I have been intimately close for years."

Giacometti looked at us like he was watching a bar fight over a game of darts.

"The Fall Into Freedom... that is what you should call the painting. Yes. I think it should be titled... The Fall Into Freedom! OR... you can simply cut the damn thing up and mend the roof with it. Has anyone enough fool's sense to notice the puddle on the floor?"

By this time water was dripping steadily from the roof. Drops of water slapped me on my cheek and continued dripping. I always knew the hole was there but since it rained so seldom I put off climbing unto the roof and covering the hole with duck tape.

In what seemed like seconds, the rain found its strength and fell hard like ropes of diamonds out of the sky and fell through the hole like a pouty faucet.

I shoved the brush's bucket under the drippings and moved the floored paintings to the side and then I put the 'Fall Into Freedom', aka the *Adam and Eve* close to the fan to speed up its drying.

The lights flickered. The storm yelled and slapped everything electric off and on twice. The voices of my ghostly colleagues laughed and drunkenly stirred around under my skin. My eyes glassed over the room filled with lazy drying color. The floor was silky smooth like the body of water circling the deck of the Titanic all glazed and deep in wonderings; prisms of things not seen and full of longing. A thrilling pulse went through me. My nights of painting always had an angel's blessing. I looked back around the studio and noticed my colleagues had made themselves disappear. They left like birds before a storm.

Quickly the skies fell apart and a thousand stars peeked through the one tiny window at the far end of the studio telling me the storm was just passing through.

Then, out of nowhere, I heard a scraping clangorous sound from somewhere outside. The noise was like the edge of a steel knife; the blade hurt my ears. My eyes tightened. I couldn't look. A grating sound of metal scraping against concrete shoved all my happiness aside.

Snowplows with huge wheels wearing chained bonnets had pushed through the studio walls in my head. Cinder blocks fell and tripped over each other crushing gallons of my color. The spillage was heavy and slippery. A cloud of dust and ash thickened and spread over the murky colored quicksand. Paint in a slow frenzy poured out and swam into each other quickly for support. But they lost their substance and drowned in a sea of muddy gray with only a few tiny splotches of color here and there holding on to their integrity. I stood there so powerless and in terror… my masterpieces.

*

"Are you ok lady?"

Everything outside my head shook quickly. My eyes

tightened themselves. I slouched deeper into the car seat and cringed in tortuous contortions.

A plow clearing the parking lot piled my studio to the side. When I opened my eyes, I saw a huge metal blade that covered my entire windshield. I could barely see anything above it.

I thought for sure no one knew I was in the car. My friends, my family, people who knew me, they were out there behind the glass windshield and mounds of snow.

The plow's driver threw his weight on the heavy lever and the plow clutched and shrieked to a halt. A voice hollered: "Are you ok lady? Do you need a tow?"

My head's voice began to quarrel with me. The quarreling tightened my breath. *I want to go home, I just want to go home for just one night. I want to forget about my mom and the dementia for just one more day.*

I tightly closed my eyes again but everything inside began running in circles as fast as it could like a rabid dog chasing his own tail. Disturbed by my failure to trick my head into returning, cordial indignation was all I could offer the terrorists of my fate and the gods who seemed to be juggling frivolously the misfortunes in my life.

I waved at the plow's voice and signaled I was fine.

Inside the car it was forcefully warm and dry as dust. The windshield looked like the top of the ocean to a fish's eye. The wipers returned to clearing the wet mess.

I drove in the snows darkness back to my mother's house.

*

It was easier this time to push in the front door and walk into the house. The duck tape that was originally used to secure the doors' closing, lost its grip. I had no energy left. Balls of scrunched octopi from the morning's ambush scattered the floor looking as if they were waiting for an apology.

My duffel bag was waiting in front hall where I had left it the night before. Everything was dark and for the life of me I couldn't remember where the light switch was located. A large window brought in just enough of the outside to clear a walking path down the steps. My bag, pulled by its shoulder strap, jumped from step to step, following me from behind.

I looked around for some place to fit. The room was packed with furniture. Provincials, bruised Chippendales and Bohemian chic mixed together unfavorably as if they've been arguing and suddenly stopped talking the second I walked into the room. A baby grand piano and an organ were in there somewhere, camouflaged in the clutter.

Scattered around the room were stacks of boxes and fat bags stuffed with projects that moved about the house over the years; projects that aged while waiting for their purpose. Boxes on top lived with the delusion that something inside of them would be uncovered and considered useful once again.

On the far end of the room was a pool table piled with runaway chattels like refugees in a small boat on the Pacific. I remember when the pool table was actually a pool table with a terrible slant, which confused its balls and angered its players.

All the walls were furnished and there was no floor, just a combination of rugs on top of rugs and shags on Orientals. The Orientals didn't seem to mind. Everything was dubiously placed yet collectively they all seemed to be part of a strange alliance.

The room was quiet. The heater clicked in and blew its hot air from an overhead duct into my face. I stood there for a time; my eyes absorbed everything as if for the first time.

Directly in front of me was the couch. No one could overlook its presence. A leather couch cut in sections with boxes drunkenly stacked on its cushions. The center section had barely a sliver of space for someone to sit if they were inclined to. What little energy I had, I pushed my butt into the space. The couch moved a bit at first, the cushions took different sides leaving my ass hanging in the middle.

I was beginning to feel one with the clutter: a balance of disproportion. My thoughts fell over each other and whined heavily in my lap. There was no place to rest the day, to forget. As it was, the day just stood there in front of my face.

God must have had something up his sleeve because everything looked too bad to be permanent.

I unclipped one earring, held it out in front of my slumped body and looked inside the hoop's circle with one eye. The hoop scanned the room until the earring's hole was filled with a suitable visual distraction that would take me someplace other than where I was sitting at the moment.

With my index finger and thumb I moved the earring around as if I were focusing the lens of the camera. At one point I found an interesting collage of colors. Inside the hoop was a thick textured color of green like foliage and through it a sweep of blue as in a sky but unlike God's sky. The image grew into a massive circle containing what seemed to be an endless curving gallery; the walls filled with great paintings. Groups of people stood appreciating and examining the art.

My eye stayed in the hoop's circle and noticed a tiny part of color that when I squinted, resembled a painting that looked much like my Adam and Eve. The painting I left in my studio...

My dear, dear *Adam and Eve.*

10.
THE FIRST ADAM AND EVE

I remember I had bought that canvas several months ago at the Salvation Army. It had been a good buy. The painting was 36 by 48 inches. It had appeared to be layered with a number of paintings that the previous artist had abandoned. That's what made it so appealing. I was familiar with this layered concept. Most of my own paintings had been painted over a number of times primarily for economic reasons but nevertheless they could be considered part of a noteworthy movement that I often refer to as *layer'ism.*

LAYERISM

[Every painting has the tormented
soul of the artist embedded in its canvas
even after it's been re-painted, primed
or cut up to patch the holes in a roof.
It never goes away. It is part of the
canvased painting forever.]

The painting had many lives in its layers. I felt it had traveled through mountainous landscapes and laid in gardens where young buds were pushing their way into their bloom. I am sure it had caressed many breasts lying on rich velvet couches and stood in deserts where wildebeest and zebras walked slowly in the jellied heat of a hot orange afternoon. This was a good purchase indeed.

First, the top surface needed to be painted with primer. It was an ungodly mess to cover. A crowd of women's heads, maybe forty, had been stacked in rows on top of each other like mangos at a market. The women were made up in oranges and yellows that they had taken from the desert's hot summer; they outlined themselves in black. Their over-sized almond shaped eyes followed me around my studio as if they were begging me to shroud them in Zinsser's BullsEye primer, possibly for religious purposes. I really didn't know.

My mentor had once told me, "Artists must paint an Adam and Eve before they die and a Crucifixion before they see the truth. It is part of the journey."

He was a Jewish man, a painter and writer, a photographer and an intellectual. He was an extremely serious fellow who would read books about the holocaust on beautiful sunny afternoons to clear his mind of paint and prose and red grapes. He was my mentor, my delicious polar counterpart. We were an item in the artist community and very seldom were seen apart from each other.

"Artists stand on the edge focused on the fear of falling but also with a terrified impulse to throw themselves off the cliff. Man has a choice. An artist sees the vulgarity and authenticity inside those choices in the face of his canvas. It is a horrifying depth of responsibility." I tried to turn away at first, tightened my smile away from his seriousness, but truth be said, I openly fell into the arms of his every word. My temperature warmed looking up into his dark black eyes, his lips moistened every message as if it were intended only for me to hear.

"And of course, the Crucifixion is the battle in our minds. Crucifying the ego. The balance of losing oneself and at the same time staying connected with one's presence. Very important for a serious artist as yourself." He gave me everything he had and everything I needed.

I left my life in Chicago years ago and moved to California to live with my mentor in his hut; originally a small bathhouse built in the 1900's. The bathhouse, a tiny box that I respectfully referred to as 'the hut' was loosely constructed with thin wood planks and glue. If a strong gale cared to, it could have blown our hut across the world like matchsticks in the wind. To our great fortune, the winds paid us little attention. The only door was a red worn wool blanket nailed to the top of its conventional framed opening. Loose bricks kept its hem to the ground. It worked quite well keeping the hut's insides from pouring out.

The living space inside was modest and small in its size - a bit under 250 square feet and furnished little beyond a bed, a small desk with a typewriter and an armed chair. Attached somehow to the walls were bookcases whose crowded shelves indicated that my mentor denied it nothing. A sink and motel-sized refrigerator topped with two stove burners hugged the corner. We had hardly an option but to paint outside under an overhang that lipped the building. Wisteria, clematis, canary eyes and trumpet creepers tightly walled in our working space. Long sheets of clear plastic seamed together with clothespins were added for protection from the cold nights and culturally starved raccoons.

We painted intensely and passionately far into the night. On one side, my mentor painted on canvases with thick, palette knife strokes that were complicated, esoteric and beautiful; part of a series he called *Rock-Water-Sky*. On the other side, just feet away, I painted a magical world brimming with color, alive and fanciful. The space was small for creating such diverse masterpieces. Stepping back from our canvases, we often bumped and became absorbed into the parts of each other.

Local philosophers, inventors and dreamers, disheveled looking characters, visited the hut often late into the nights. For hours our visitors circled around theories over wine and cheese and refuted published philosophies found in professor'ed books. They brought their inventions and tested their applications with only one small fire that I can remember. They talked over each other, argued passionately and laughed loudly late into the night. The Marlboros and Camels, the Newports and cannabis paid no mind and simply absorbed the air collectively enjoying the flavors of each other.

I was living in eternal happiness, that an everlasting unbridled security, a blessedness or blindness of sorts.

I was at home until my mentor's death - his heart just stopped.

My hair still rises all over my body when I think of him.

[I moved away from the hut to a
cinder block warehouse with no vines.
The new studio was stronger. I took
the crowded shelved books with me.]

*

The phone rang. I clipped the earring back on my ear and stumbled to the phone quickly. Its ring hurt my ears.

"Suzka, this is your mother. Where have you been? I'd been calling the house."

"I... I just got in mom."

"How's the house? Is everything ok? How'd you get in? I hope you didn't use the front door. You know I spent a lot of time duck-taping it shut. Tell me you didn't use that door." Her words were sharp and clear.

"Everything is ok mom. It's terribly late. You're in the hospital for God's sake. Why are you calling me?"

"It's your father. You need to talk to him. He's making me crazy. You need to give him a piece of my mind."

"Father?"

"Yes, your father... he's in the bathroom. Don't put him on the phone 'cause he won't talk to me but he'll talk to you. Just go and talk to him."

I didn't know what to say. My father was not in the bathroom. He died seven years ago.

Willem deKooning died that same year.

11.
THE A.O.P.
(Aged Oaks Pavilion)

I returned to the hospital the next morning.

"Day took her an hour ago, justa after lunch... spaghetti anda one meataball da size of a pea. Didn't day tell you ada nurses' desk?" Josephine reported.

She caught me off-guard. "Wwwwhat...?" I stood there motionless and pressed my eyes hard toward the yellow drawn curtains that veiled my mother absence.

"What did you say?"

"You mother... she slept good last night. All doze bad drugs left her to sleep alone."

My legs took me across the room carefully as if they were walking me through minefields of ignited chatter. The curtains that divided my mother from Josephine were short for the overgrown room and respectfully offered only a veiled sense of privacy. But Josephine bent her voice and slid it under the curtains' hem.

"Just a lil' while ago, two mens put your mother's body on a gurney, covered her up with two flimsy blankets and wheeled her out."

Josephine believed there were only two choices when gurney'd out of a room. You were either sent to a nursing home like The Aged Oaks Pavilion or you were sent to the morgue two floors below ground level.

I didn't care to answer.

"Are you closa to your mother? It's good when a mother has girl childrens. I have only boy childrens. They live far away... except for Albert. He lives closa. He's a policeman. He saves many peoples and digs out bodies from da rivers. Da Des Plaines River is a good one for that. My son's a good boy he is. His wife is much more lucky getting him than he is for sure."

I looked out the window and squinted through the hard light. The sun was flat against my eyes. I just stood there with my arms loosely folded against my chest looking at nothing. I had neither the time nor the presence of mind to take in any additional information. Maybe it was a curious numbness that had overcome me. I kept my thoughts to a whisper afraid Josephine might hear. With no response coming from my side of the curtain, Josephine returned to the subject of my mother.

"Are you taking your mother home? She's..."

Josephine knew my mother wasn't going home.

I really didn't care to answer but I knew the only way to stop Josephine's reckless chatter was to sacrifice a quick answer.

"She's going to The Aged Oaks Pavilion." *...period!*

"Ohhhh..." she timidly replied with conversation-stopping disappointment even though she was fully aware of what the answer would be before she asked the question.

I started to look for any possessions my mother might have left behind; clues perhaps confirming my mother was here minutes before they took her to The Aged Oaks nursing home.

My legs bent, my body slowly rested on the edge of her bed.

On the bed tray a yellow sheet of paper, folded four times and hand pressed to deepen its folds. On top read "To Suzka – My Daughter."

The scribbled lettering underlined daughter eight times. It had all the makings of a testimony, a final request just lying there for me to execute. Not that I didn't hear all her requests for as long as I can remember. This folded paper was obvious and unavoidable. My life was about to change.

My brain was processing all the possible scenarios with screwed-up endings. It was already a long day. My head was bursting; my mouth was like a dirty shoe. I didn't want to be here. I wanted to get back to work. I missed my life. I missed my studio, Picasso and color, wet glorious color. And my hands, my hands were shamefully clean. They had no color, no paint under the nail parts and stuck in the corners of their moons. I tucked them deep in my pockets to hide my shame.

Flashing before my eyes were all those unpainted, controversially inspired masterpieces that I would have created if I were home. And what would come of my paints and my canvases waiting to be great pieces of art? I slaughtered myself with exasperation. I'm too old to start over, I'm too young to end it all and too damn poor not to worry.

This was not going to be good but who was to blame? To accuse my mother, the gods, the circumstances would be selfish, blind, deaf and simply stupid. My life's legs and hands were pulling me in the all sorts of disjointed directions.

I set myself down on the bed and dug into my purse for my glasses. My hand ran away from me - fingers frantically formed a search party looking for an old lost pack of cigarettes at the bottom, in the corners or maybe in one of the side pockets. I needed a friend more than eyeglasses. But it had been over five years since smoking and I broke-up. I can't say it was mutual. We had one of those tragic endings. I walked out with no warning, no sign but a promise to my friend, my cigs that I would return. We would meet again on my ninety-fifth birthday. The promise made me feel better.

Final goodbyes are so devastating and cruel. I'm not cruel.

The paper was filled with writing, underlining, stars, crosses and instructional doodles. Each item coded in its importance.

----> TO SUZKA MY DAUGHTER
BRING THESE ITEMS TO ME.
I NEED EVERYTHING ON THIS LIST!
#1 -> A SIX PACK OF ENSURE, THE BUTTER PECAN
#2. MY RED CRYSTAL ROSARY (IN THE BLUE KIMONO POCKET)
#3. A BLACK SUIT AND MY ITALIAN SLING-BACK HIGH HEELS.
#4. BRING MY PEACH BLOUSE HANGING IN THE LAUNDRY ROOM,
A SLIP, A FRESH GARMENT, PANTYHOSE AND A BRASSIERE
#5. AND THE HALL'S COUGH DROPS + FOUR RAIN BONNETS.
BRING ME THE SMALL SACRED HEART STATUE
BETWEEN THE MARY AND JOSEPH
SALT-N-PEPPER SHAKERS ON THE
KITCHEN COUNTER NEXT TO THE TOASTER.

AND... <u>TWO</u> BOTTLES OF <u>CAMPHO-PHONIQUE</u> ...AND

*** BRING <u>SEVEN</u> ZIP-LOCK BAGS OF CANDIES***
(MAKE THREE OF THEM SUGARLESS)
V
X <u>VIOLET, YOUR MOTHER</u>

*

It was about two o'clock in the afternoon when I walked into The Aged Oaks nursing home carrying two large bags containing her listed items and one succulent, a gift from my sister in California. It was a one-story square building, red brick with white trim. The entrance was under a canopy that extended two car lengths into a circled driveway. The lobby was carpeted wide in a cut looped pile with tiny oak leaves. The decor was outdated colonial - the walls were covered in flowering paper that looked as if it was personally brought here by one of those early traders voyages ago. The paper tragically held in a strange collection of odors. Straight across the lobby was an opened archway into the linoleumed side of the building.

An older lady sat at a wood table with Victorian shapely legs; the 'check-in' desk for all incoming visitors. Oddly, the table was sitting halfway into the opening to the corridor; an apparent precaution to block strays from wandering in off the street and running around willy-nilly in the halls. For whatever reason, it was impossible to walk past this little volunteer without being questioned.

Looking over her glasses, she caught my presence and stopped me from squeezing past her. "Hello dearie. Welcome to the Aged Oaks Nursing Pavilion. Is there someone here you would like to visit today?"

There was no guessing as to what this lady was up to. Under her pearls was a tight-lipped mama. She looked like the type who came to work early, when it was dark, before any staff workers arrived in order to push her desk half way into the archway without being detected; yes, pushing it into a position that would stop anyone from walking past her without verification. She looked relentless, checking for undocumented visitors as if this was Tijuana's port of entry. No one was going to cross on her watch - not without her confirmation. She had a sinister side for sure.

Her general appearance was her disguise. She had a smiling head, lacquered in purpose that bobbled out of a turtleneck sweater as if it were spring-coiled to her body. She wore half glasses chained to hang that gave her a more qualified look of importance. Baby pearl earrings softened her czarist manner and added just enough Americana-n-apple-pie needed for this position.

I laid the one bag on the floor and set the succulent on the czar's desk. The air in the room gasped. I felt the oak leaves in the carpet flipped themselves over. A coldness hit my face. The little lady froze. Her eyes left her papers and jumped on the succulent. I swear that juicy plant looked up at me and winced. She raised the succulent carefully in the air and strategically positioned a notepad under its elevated bottom. Then slowly she lowered the plant. Its landing was deliberate and dead-on.

"My mother Violet was brought here about an hour ago. Can you tell me her room number?"

From ear to ear, her denture'd smile loosely rested on her face. She appeared friendly enough but serious.

"Is she a new resident here at The Aged Oaks? I don't recognize the name." She said oh so cheerfully.

She looked down at a paper filled with columned names - residents' names apparently. "We do have a Frank Schavzak... but he's not a Violet. Hmmmm, could your mother be Vera? Here's a Vafi. Hmm, I know

Vafi..." She pivoted her chin on her index finger. Her dentures clapped down on the corner of her lip. After a few seconds, she looked up at me and moved her head side to side. "But she's not your mother. She's Chinese. Your mother is not a Chinese woman is she?"

I had to remind myself to stay calm, she's only doing her job, the best she can... *to keep the handles moving on the sausage machine.* Words my friend Gulley Jimson often told me: *Everyone, at one time or another has to keep the handles moving on the sausage machine. And where would we all be without sausage.* I swear, standing at the little blocker's desk, I smelled the tiny scent of salami.

"No, my mother's name is Violet, like the flower."

"I have a Lilly... Lilies are pretty flowers too."

My head's voice with no control on my part, was begging for some relief. *Oh God, just give her the room number. And for God's sake, don't bring out the Home's floor plan or the pamphlets with the list of all your social activities. No, no, no. We're tired. I'm tired. My succulent is tired. We've been through a lot today. For God's sake, have mercy on us both and just give me a number... ANY FRICKIN' NUMBER!*

I so wanted to tell her... *Listen, what do you got here, 50 rooms tops, I'm bi-numeral and fluent in both roman and English numbers, one through fifty. I can do this.*

"Just one minute, you wait right here honey." The little Czar walked into another room behind her desk; the room that contained the A.O.P. pamphlets and the paid office staff.

I looked around the lobby carefully as to not arouse and suspicion and checked if anyone was watching. A choice was made. I would risk being reported to the home's authorities of my crossing over to the linoleum'ed side. Quickly I grabbed my bags, the succulent and scooted my way around the desk and into the hallway. I was now considered one of the A.O.P.'s undocumented immigrant visitors.

12.
THE LINOLEUM'ED SIDE OF THE A.O.P.

The other side was where residents lived in little rooms they shared with strangers. Muffled music came from small black boxes nailed to the wall's corners playing *'Spanish Eyes'* - a popular selection from a musical soirée of institutional tunes. The music slid down the wall-to-wall linoleum sideways.

At first sight was an enormous ornate bird aviary. It was about ten feet wide and towering up to a sizable bubbled skylight at the ceiling. In the center of the aviary was a tree, a living tree filled with canaries, finches, button quails and twinspots. The tree was packed with multi-level perches, bird sized ladders, resting shelves with living flowers and vine'd plants. Wild vegetation mixed around the ripened debris making it a suitable home for the tiny creatures. Tree leaves provided little vistas. You lost sight of where you were for a moment. It was a birdcage sanctuary like no other I had ever seen.

The hall appeared empty except for a large dark man who was wheeling an empty wheelchair toward me. He was wearing the institutional whites and walked with a lisp. A Philippine gentleman with a wide moon face and big teeth that spread themselves far apart like the islands of his home. When he got closer, I noticed a silver nameplate pinned on his jacket. It read Horny.

"Excuse me, uhhh... Horny...Mr. Horny I am..." My thoughts ran outside of my control.

"Oh no, zat's my firz name. My baptize name is Horrrr-ace Nacapuy. Everyone here shorts it to Horny."

"Wow. That's...interesting. Well... Horny, I'm looking for my mother. She's a short sweet lady about this height, sitting down of course. Her name is Violet. Do you know what room she's in?"

"I juz took her to room numbrrr eight. Right in dahh." Horny pointed to a room just a few steps back. He shook his head from side to side expanding his smile even wider.

"Your mahDa is a berry sweet lady and very exzay-ted. She oppered me many bahgz of cahndy if I would keep on going and tak her out da door, down da street and to her home dat chee said was not far from here. She told me not to worry cuz she would reward me well she said."

He laughed, a full and genuine belly laugh that pushed everything up into his chest. His laugh opened his mouth showing all the pearled islands.

"She went to beggin', promising me many zings." His eyes disappeared in a squeeze. "Cheez'a funny lady."

"Yes, she's a funny lady. Thanks Horny."

I watched Horny bobble down the hall, laughing in rhythm to the institution's 'Spanish Eyes' – an image that was soon interrupted by the climate around me.

My eyes started to burn a bit. My nose desperately tried to close down entry to all foreign odors from entering. Old urines embarrassingly apologized for their accidents. They tried to cover up their piddle odors with bouquets of Pine Sol and lavender. The linoleum just shined it away.

*

My mother was already sitting on her bed, dressed. She did not look happy.

"Don't leave me here!" She bladed her stare, the sharpest point laid at the center of my daughter-ness. She spat out those words clearly in spite of her clamped down dentures.

"When are we going home?" she repeated every twenty minutes or when there was a dent in the present conversation.

The room had two beds. My mother's bed was closest to the door. A woman younger than her occupied the bed by the window. She looked to be about in her late 60's; a vanilla woman, Protestant looking, large in stature and compacted. Even in bed, you knew this woman had no curves or angles. Her hair was short bobbed and boxed to her head. She complimented the room's decor as if she were a piece of its furniture.

The room ate up all the sound. My mother sat on her bed with her back to the window side. She was fully dressed, bus-ready.

I directed my attention to the woman on the other side of the room.

"Hello. My name is Suzka. I don't know if you have met my mother, her name is Violet. She'll be your roommate for a couple of days."

My head was stuck. It refused to turn and give my mother all of my face. I made her ten-day stay at the home sound like an overnight Tupperware party.

She heard me. I felt her stare at the back of my head calling me a liar.

“Don’t leave me here. When are we going home?”

The lady roommate said very little and chopped off the better parts of her story. "My name was Beulah but everyone calls me Bea." – that was all the information she offered.

The room was stagnantly quiet except for the rain. It lasted all day, harder and consistent like the ringing of a telephone with no one to answer on the other end. Its sound slammed against the window and kept ringing and slamming and ringing and slamming.

I tried to help my mother get settled into her new space. Bea paid us no attention and guarded herself from falling into any conversation by staring into a book. Her eyes were watering but not with tears, just naturally watering. They never moved like they should have if they were reading in honesty. She must have found the goings on in her head to be more interesting than the book she held in her hand and more entertaining than my mother or myself.

“Don’t leave me here. When are we going home?”

I laid out the listed items my mother requested on the bed and hung her black suit in a side tall metal closet. On top of the closet I placed the succulent.

My mother defiantly remained sitting on the edge of her bed. Her eyes closed themselves but remained staring at me from the inside - the gift God gave mothers.

"Where's the Campho?" Her focused anger broke.

"It's here, it's here someplace."

I couldn't help but notice that lying on her bed was a remote control of familiarity, the remote control from home. "And why do you have this remote with you? Where did it come from? You know it won't work here in your room, mom. This remote is for the TV back home and will ONLY work on the TV back at the house."

"Never you mind." Violet grabbed it out of my hand and threw it up in the air, over her head and screamed when she missed catching it on its way down.

She looked at me with waxed eyes. I brushed it off. Then with both her fists she grabbed the rain bonnets, her gloves, her hairnet, and tubes of her vitamin skin lotions and tossed them all in the air as if it were confetti.

“When are we going home?”

I was paralyzed to respond.

“Don’t you leave me here.”

At this point, I could only watch.

She continued her outburst and propelled her girdle, her brassieres, the cough drops, the bananas, bottles of Ensure and a pope-blessed rosary, each time tossing them harder and with more force and in each shot her aim got closer to the ceiling.

The tossed Ensure came down first and torpedoed into a spin missing me by barely an inch. I jumped back in fear of getting hit. That's when I fell against the metal closet behind me, slamming its door shut. If it weren't for my rubber'd bottom boots, I would have slid down hitting the floor hard. She then grabbed her shoes, the Italian heels, her Sergio Rossi for God sake, and propelled them in the air with both hands as hard as she could. They went fast and high, hit the ceiling and crashed broken on the linoleum floor. The sound triggered something inside of her. Her face changed. My mother surprised herself and smirked.

It was euphoric and distorted all at the same time. My mother appeared elated at first and at the same time desperately determined. She frantically grabbed anything remaining that was not grounded. Looking up and using more force than she thought she had, she threw things high and hard as if she was trying to break through the ceiling's plaster, to crack an opening wide for the sun to come in and rescue her, pulling her out of some underground prison.

In slow motion, in the final desperate toss to the merciful gods, my mother's eyes fell on the sole surviving object saved from her rampage - a pitcher half filled of water sitting on a side table. Before I could get to her, she gripped the pitcher with both hands, lowered it between her knees and hurled it to the ceiling. The pitcher hit the ceiling. Its water met my mother on the way down.

The rain outside kept ringing. I couldn't help but notice that Bea remained motionless. She barely blinked during the madness that just swept through the room. She remained cemented in holding her book through the entire storm. How could anyone fake reading in the middle of such bedlam? My head's concerns bounced back and forth visiting both sides of the room. *Jesus, could anyone be that drugged? Maybe she's in a coma... or, or maybe she's... dead! Oh my God, I hope we didn't kill her.*

Suddenly my mother began to hiccup. Her wet hair jumped with every bout and spasm. Her face was shiny wet. I put a towel around her shoulders and absorbed most of the water. She looked up at me as if she wanted to slap me silly and I wasn't sure why. Maybe she wasn't sure either.

Then she did the strangest thing. She scooted off the bed, got on her hands and knees and delicately picked up every piece of clothing and every tiny bead from the floor. She collected the crystals and placed them in her pocket and carefully folded all her clothes on to the bed as if she were a new bride.

I looked at my mother, but she turned away.

A few minutes later, she looked at me and raised her fingers in the air and motioned for me to come close.

"Come here. Come closer." My mother's eyes were as big as baby onions. I leaned in closer to hear the little bride's words.

"Suzka, I want you to talk to your father. He's driving me crazy."

*

Horny walked in shortly after hearing the commotion and immediately began mopping up the water on the floor with a towel he grabbed from the bathroom. Behind him a small crowd of curious residents stood close like a bunch of bananas on an animated spy mission.

A little man clothed in oversized flannel was the first to enter the room. His face was like a cod, his color like a new potato. He was completely bald and had no hair whatsoever except for the back of his hands.

"Is she ok? He asked.

"Yes, of course. She's fine. My mother is fine. We're just airing out a few things."

The little bald man looked down and stared strangely at my boots. I said quickly, "Oh no, no, that's paint. I'm a painter *(pause)* an artist. I get a little messy when I paint sometimes *(pause and looking for some understanding).*

"Believe me. It's red paint." I knew where he was going with his thoughts. "Really, it's not blood. It's just dried paint."

The entire group as well as my mother seemed to be spending an unfavorable amount of time looking down at my boots, except for Bea of course, "...red paint with a little bit of orange paint specs on the sides. See, right here." The home's residents showed no signs of believing anything I said.

No one said a word for the longest time.

“Oh for God’s sake, if it were blood it would be a much darker red and purplish… and maroon around the edges. Come on now, I seriously don't see how any normal person can think that would be blood."

I don't know why I continued talking. I told myself… *Stop talking. For God’s sake, stop talking.*

The little bald man kept looking at me. I didn't notice that I was noticing until he looked back up at me and said, "Pitiful." *Was he talking to me?*

Behind him, a lady wearing a chenille robe and bunny slippers burst into tears with no accompanying sound. I smiled at her out of pure benevolence.

"Everything is just fine. I am so sorry we disturbed you. This is my mother Violet. She is just moving in."

The lady's face shrunk to a shelled walnut except for a tiny button nose that was pink.

The bald man turned his head around and reported his evaluation of the situation to the small crowd behind him.

"She's a new one".

The air circling the group changed. The crowd began chanting in choir’d whispers.

"Ohhh... she’z new."

The little man could not sustain his interest.

"Time to go. It's Wheel of Fortune night in the dining room. Move. Show’s over, I gotta go.”

The man turned abruptly bumping and pushing aside the other curious residents. "Move, move over, let me through." The crowd turned around and followed.

13.
WHEEL OF FORTUNE

Violet went to church twice a day; once in the morning for 7:00 mass and again at 6:30 at night. It was not that she a religious zealot. She never pushed her beliefs on anyone or solicited lost souls. She was Catholic. Her life was wrapped in the mesmerizing rituals of the Catholic magic and mystery. She talked to all the blessed ghosts in her heart; the Jesuses, all the Marys and the Abrahams. She told God what she needed.

"I ask God to help and give me a sign. If God is home, He answers. If God is not home, he tells me to handle things on my own. God knows He has enough to do. It's ok with God."

But at 6:30 pm Violet was religiously devoted to a nighttime televangelist. His followers called him SayJack. Bishop SayJack was a small, suited, unassuming man who read from the Holy Wheel and talked of bankruptcy, wild cards and trips to a promise-land, a winning resort in Cabo, all expenses paid. Sista' Vanna was his assistant, an attractive blonde woman with a wide, fixed, billboard smile. She wore soft chiffon gowns and floated across an altar staged with neon green boxed squares. The Bishop's sacred message was hidden in letters found behind the chosen boxes.

At 6:30 everything stopped. Violet would sit on the edge of the sofa, push her knees up against the cluttered end table that was only a few feet from the television and turned on SayJack. She then made the sign of attention and wiggled her glasses, readjusting their position. On her lap she had a spiral ring tablet filled with scribbled information lost in its importance. She pressed up the volume button on the remote and tucked it under her arm.

The televangelist just finished the preliminary introductions and was about to address his congregation and contestants. He spoke in letters to all his devoted followers everywhere. Contestants called out consonants and bought vowels hoping to make the Bishop's squares light up. Chosen squares illuminated themselves in Windex blue. Sista' Vanna gently tapped on the chosen square's shoulder, asking the square to reveal itself. Bells would ring and the skies would open up. The chosen square would silently scream, exposing its letter. *I'm a D, I'm a D. Yes, I'm a glorious D.*

With just a few letters revealing themselves, nervous believers everywhere tried desperately to guess the Bishop's message. Sounds a bit weird but most religious cults are weird.

cult (kəlt) *noun*

– a system of misplaced excessive admiration directed toward a particular person or object; synonyms: obsession, (game) mania, movement

The service finished at 6:58. I'd call her at 7:03.

"Mom, ya got'em?" A game we played.

"Yes, yes. Let me see here. There was Fly Me To The Moonshine, that was the first one, and then there was Venetian Blinds, then Leave Your Baggage at the Door, and then Kick It and Make It Better. I think the next one was Naked Potatoes but I can't read it clearly. My pen got stuck on the paper and stopped my writing. You know, maybe it was Laked Potatoes. The bonus one was Genocide. That I know for sure. Do you want me to repeat them?"

"No. Thanks mom. I'll call you later."

"Call me tomorrow. My number is 312-555-6..."

"I gotta go mom. I'm painting. Good night."

Click.

*

I was living in California during those days. Life was good. Mother was acting like the mother I was familiar with and mosquitos carrying diseases minded their own business. I had my own life with a small circle of like-minded friends. Greg was part of that circle. He was a friend and a colleague; a picture framer by day and musician by night. His money gig was framing.

Greg was a physically large well-rounded guy who always wore short-sleeved, buttoned-down, blue cotton shirts. He was an incredible musician, an off-the-wall percussionist who slammed his drums with jaw dropping rhythms. We worked together on a number of musical dance performances in the past.

[Remembering a time
before mosquitoes bit innocent
mothers on hot summer days and
the Fly Me To The Moonshine sting]

The bell rang in the back workroom; a huge room packed with frames, frame parts, pressing machines and lawn chairs. In the center was a large table, waist high, where Greg matted and framed local art pieces, yellowed photos, war metals and other memorabilia his customers wanted held down under glass.

Greg was wiping finger smudges off a sheet of glass he had just cut. Around the table were the regulars, the local odd balls off the street, homies that spoke in puns on a variety of unrelated subjects.

"Hi guys." I took off my shades and leaned on the large working table in the center of the room. "Just checking in."

Greg would have said hello but he already put a pun in motion and there was no way to stop its speed.

"...and he asked the bartender, *Ya got any special drinks today?* ..and the bartender said, *Yes, we have a new drink that was invented by a Gynecologist. It's a mix of Pabst Blue Ribbon and Smirnoff Vodka. We call it the Pabst Smir.*"

Uncle Pete who was not an uncle to anyone, 'upped' Greg's quip with..."That must be the same bar where a jumper cable walked in and the bartender says, *I'll serve you, but don't start anything.*"

Just then Bob jumped out of a sitting sleep and made a face like a man who had ice drop down his back. "How much time do I got on my parking. Anybody remember when I walked in here?"

Bob lived in his van. His days rotated around avoiding meter maids ticketing violators. No one answered Bob. Everyone was mindfully occupied arming themselves with pun comebacks. Bob had strong opinions.

"That new meter maid is a crazy bitch. She'd give a ticket to Mother Theresa parked in front of a bar giving out free ginger ale to sick people who needed a slug."

At the same time an old boxy Sony television talking reruns in the background politely made its way in and out of the tables discussion.

"Hey, Suzka, where ya been?"

"Around."

Mrs. Greg, an opera singer sat in a lawn chair chatting with her daughter-in-law on the phone. She gave me the five finger wave of recognition and went back to her phone conversation. Her eyes traveled alone to the one wall that was not obstructed with equipment. The wall displayed a series of art pieces created by their only grandson. The order on the wall recorded his young life. The number of pinholes in the corners of the papered art pieces gave away their age. The wall had been rearranged over the years to make room for the most current piece. Their grandson was now 18. There was no more rearranging and no more room. The collection was complete.

"Give me an S." The old Sony television's words were clearly heard in the background and made their way into the conversation without interrupting its flow.

"There is one S," said the Sony.

A blonde Sista'Vanna strolled across Sony's dusty screen and flipped one square in the line of 19 blanks. Before the blonde got to the end of the screen, I spoke.

My voice ripped the room like a pair of scissors cutting through a long fabric of silk - "Fly Me to the Moonshine."

The homies left their thoughts; Greg raised his eyes from the glass. Mrs. Greg squinted, looking closer into the television and back to me. The room's punning stopped.

After the puzzle's time expired, after exhausting all the possibilities, the contestant inside the Sony spoke slowly pausing between each word. "I'd like to solve the puzzle. FLY...ME...TO...THE... MOONSHINE."

Everyone froze in place. They first looked at the TV screen and then moved their eyes to me. No one said a word. "How'd she do that?" circled the room like an excited fly on the wharf after the squid festival.

Frankie sat back down in his chair. "Holy shit. How'd she do that?'

"She's creepy!"

"Anybody know much time I got on my parking?"

14.
THE W.O.F at the A.O.P

Every Sunday there were two activities scheduled at the same time at The Aged Oaks Pavilion - a compressed, nondenominational prayer service, held in a small room that was primarily used as a patient-doctor lounge on the Monday through Saturday days and the *Wheel of Fortune* in the main dining room with a seating capacity of three hundred.

This is good. This is very good, I told myself. *Surely this would change her attitude.* I wheeled my mother to the dining room that was set up into a mini game show studio. On the far end of the room, a white bed sheet was tacked and draped from one column to another. Perched across the top were colored clothespins holding large cards to the sheet. Blank cards. Their backs were marked with one letter, a clue to the answer in the word puzzle.

The room was full of erratic traffic. The cane'd and walk'ables rolled and wobbled around for the best position near the sheeted stage. Smells of dry parchment, rose water, medicine and a nip of Yukon Jack to wash down the meds followed.

The scents Le Baiser du Dragon and Narciso Rodriguez hovered around the stronger women. The Estee, Shalimar, L'Heure Bleue and a gaggle of others squeezed in there somehow unnoticed.

A man in the corner of the room tried to take off his sweater without losing his hair. The lady wearing the chenille robe and bunny slippers, waved at us to come closer.

Most of the room was in movement except for gridlocked section in a center isle. A rather engaging character with bulgy white eyelids stopped and stood heroically stoic without moving an inch. You would have thought he was glued to the floor. People kept rolling around him as if he were a familiar curve in an often-traveled road.

Then suddenly, a suited man with glass eyes and a nose like a badly scraped carrot began waving his fist and shouting in my face.

"What do you think you're doing? You can't just park yourself here. This is my seat. Everyone knows that. Every Sunday I sit in this exact spot at this exact time."

The agitated man looked around nervously. "And what did you do with my ascot? It is very expensive. Where is it? Where is my ascot? "

"I... I don't know where it is, I really don't." *What's an ascot?*

"I don't like that tone. You maz'well learn now girlie that we have rules around here. We have rules that everyone follows without exceptions for sassy visitors like yourself."

I was an outsider to this world. I knew to back off.

I turned my back and attention into the room hoping to find a suitable space for my mother's wheelchair and a seat for myself. A second later, I heard a loud slap. The suited man's hand was gripping the arm of my mother's wheelchair.

"Get your hands off of me you old fool." The voice was familiar... my mother. I thought we were going to have a calm evening. I told myself... *Talk to everybody, use your charm; simply try to fit in.* I was everywhere in my thoughts. But in that minute I could not stop that pitiful reaction in my head to the whole damn world and all its resident crazies. I was getting myself in the worst possible state. *Stop it.*

He persisted. My mother hit him again but this time hard with her purse knocking him nearly clear off his bullishness. The suited man let go of the chair and fell back a slight bit. A friend standing at his side held his stance; a short stout character with black hair that hid his brows; hairs that originated in the back rows of his head. He had a mustache like a seal and wore a plaid robe with proud new tags hanging on its back.

The friend tried to calm the old man and pointed to a chair a few feet away. A blue satin ascot was tied to the chairs back post.

"Oh... ok. My chair seemed to have found a more suitable place with a better view. I hope you learned your lesson little lady. Have a good day." He moved on with his friend, arm-in-arm.

A female microphone voice spoke. "Ok now. I need your attention. Everyone needs to be sitting before we can start playing the Wheel of Fortune."

The crowd started to ease themselves into the night's activities. They found their seats, stretched their legs and pushed themselves backwards to snatch a little extra floor from the people behind.

Nurse Vanna, the Wheel of Fortune hostess started the night's game. Vanna was a rather chunky moon colored girl about thirty years in age with thick black hair she pulled back and gathered in a ponytail. She wore blue-rimed eyeglasses that pinched out rhinestones on both sides. When she smiled her eyes disappeared altogether behind the glass.

"Find your seat. We need for everyone to be seated before we begin. Does everyone have a number? You can't play unless you have a number."

Hands flew in the air, hands waving little worn pieces of paper with numbers written in black marker. Everyone got a number when they first walked into the room. The numbers would determine the players order.

We could win big tonight. I had watched the Wheel of Fortune with my mother often enough this past year, more often than I wish to admit to anyone. But in my humblest opinion, I considered myself quite proficient in the wheel game world.

"Mom, I feel real good about this. We're going to win it all tonight."

I couldn't stop thinking - this would be a great way to help my mother fit in with the other residents. They would admire and respect this little lady in the morning for her quick thinking and her ingenious knowledge of the wheel.

Vanna stood on top of a short stool and shouted into the crowd. "Ok everyone. Let's begin."

In back of Vanna were fifteen cards close-pinned to the sheet; five then two then eight. The letters previously written on the reverse side were hidden. The puzzle contained three words.

"Our first puzzle is the name of a movie."

Nurse Vanna then pulled a number from a large glass bowl.

"44. Whoever has the number 44 will be the first one to guess a letter. Who has 44?"

Seven hands waved their carded numbers in the air. The cards had numbers close to 44 written in felt marker. Someone in the back yelled..."Give me a B, Vanna."

A man in front turned around, "No, no. There's no B. And you never start with a B for Christ's sake." He turned his body back to nurse Vanna while waving his hand in the air. "Give her an S. You always start with the S. Holy crap, everyone knows that."

The lady who yelled out the letter 'B' was not happy. She stood up from her chair, "I know what I'm talking about. I want a B... like in *Bye Bye Birdie*."

Another woman close to my mother leaned over and said, "Oh dear. She gave us the answer. It wasn't even her turn in the first place. Her number was 23. Do you thinks that's fair?"

My mom answered. "N. She should have said N."

Soon everyone began yelling out movies they remembered that had the letter 'B' somewhere in the title - *Breakfast at Tiffany's, To Kill a Mockingbird, Chitty Chitty Bang Bang...* The old man in the corner with the loose hair piece yelled out, *"Lolita!"*

Vanna tried to calm the group. She surrendered and overturned the random letters. The yellowed sheets of paper spelled out... B I R D S O F P A R A D I S E .

I must be on another planet. What in the hell is going on around here. I leaned down to my mother. "Birds of Paradise is not a movie. It's a flower for God's sake, it's a flower."

A lady sitting in front with a pug face and soaked in lavender toilet water snapped at me.

"It is too a movie. I remember seeing the 'Birds of Paradise' with Anne Margaret and my late husband. Why are you trying to cause problems?"

The little bald man in the oversized flannel, whom I had met earlier, turned his head to the small group of serious gamers. "She's a troublemaker that one. Just look at her boots. They got blood on 'em."

A few started yelling. "Sit down. You're stopping the game. Why are you trying to ruin everything? Sit down already.“

“She'z a trouble maker that one."

My mother pulled at my arm. I leaned over.

"Suzka, are you sure Birds of Paradise is a flower?"

I tried to explain myself from a distance. Vanna was not happy with me. She avoided my presence.

After a disturbing hour and a half of misspelled titles and countless game rule violations, I wheeled my mother out into the hall. "I know we could have won big-time mom, but these people just don't play fair. They make up their own rules that make no sense whatsoever. This place pisses me off."

"But Suzka, I could swear Burt Lancaster was in The Birds of Paradise...and Myrna Loy?"

We wheedled down the corridor together. Not much more could be said. I stopped at the bird sanctuary in order to lose sight of our losses. My mother sat there watching the wonderful creatures and whistling to them. At the end of their conversations, she stood up from her chair, placed her hand on her heart and began to sing.

"Oh, say, can you see by the dawn's early light. What so proudly we hailed at the twilight's last gleaming. Whose broad stripes and bright stars through the perilous fight, o'er the ramparts we watched were so gallantly streaming... And the rockets' red glare, the bombs bursting in air, gave proof through the night that our flag was still there. O say, does that star spangled banner yet wave... O'er the land of the free and the home of the brave." When Violet finished singing she sat back down into the chair.

"Did you know that Bea was married to a black man and lived on a cattle ranch in Minnesota? They have no children." How in the hell did my mother come up with this idea.

[On that day in California the
Annual Tournament of Roses Parade
was drenched in heavy rain
for the first time in 51 years.]

When I returned the next morning to the Aged Oaks two things were brought to my attention. First, according to my mother, a woman visited her after the morning breakfast and told her she had a beautiful voice. Second, we were banned from the dining room on all Sunday's Wheel of Fortune nights.

My mother never did leave the residents with the impression of being clever, if anything they pitied her for having an unruly daughter.

I packed my mother and her ten-day accouterments in the car. But before we could officially leave, she needed to thank everyone as if they were the servicing crew on the Regal Princess cruise ship. She had eleven bags of candy to give away – three were sugarless.

"We have to wait for Horney. I think he starts to work about 9 o'clock."

"Mom, that's ten hours from now."

She quickened her thinking and brushed aside any acknowledgement of timing. "Ok. Let's go home."

My mother was wrapped in the impatience that people wear in the final hours of a long cruise.

15.
DAY ELEVEN

We walked into the house together. Without notice my mother left my side and scurried to the corner room. She moved like a leaf rolling in the wind. Her feet hurried fast and kept their balance. I followed at my own pace. I wasn't sure what to expect. My mother and I were now committed roommates now. I wasn't sure she realized I would be staying.

The corner room was filled with a warm sun that melted the edges of the day. She looked around wide-eyed almost surprised, looking in wonder as if she had walked into a large garden where every flower was in its fullest bloom. Leaves moved close to the window, the sun winked at her from behind. I couldn't help but follow her around the room. It was as if I were watching a small girl at her first day of school.

My mother plopped her purse on the couch and deflated her body into its cushions.

I stood in the margins as she ran her fingers through her hair like a rota-tiller loosening compacted roots and weeds from the hard soil. There was no sweet-talkin' comb that could have completed this job without some serious resistance. Those hairs were styled and pinned in place, trained not to move for decades. Even between washings, they knew their place. But now, without notice, they were freed from their lacquered hold.

Hundreds of bobby pins were uprooted and tossed across the room. Some hit the wall others nose-dived into the carpet. Lifting both her arms head-high in the air, my mother scratched her scalp excessively releasing every single strand – a pardon after a fifty-year sentence. After all her hairs ran out into the free world, she straightened the eye glasses on her nose and pushed herself back into the sofa. Turning her full head toward me, she spoke.

"Now that feels better!"

I never saw my mother with her hair... out... and about like that. This was radical, a subversive move on her part. I was flabbergasted. She looked like some damn fool angel that didn't even know the name of God.

Unsure of what to think, I slowly lowered my body to sitting. Half my butt landed on the sofa's cushioned edge. My mother, the woman the world called Violet with the lacquered-lavender French twist, had she gone mad?

My eyes never left the face of this strange person in front of me.

Cautiously, I leaned over to her, extending my head out slightly, barely an inch, slow and with trepidation, as you would if you were about to pet a friend's new pound rescued pit bull. I forfeited thinking and opened my mouth slowly.

"Uh... Can I get you something to drink?"

It was a respectful two hours close to five. Thoughts of alcohol seemed reasonable and warranted, considering the circumstances. A drink was the first thought that popped up in my head. I knew my mother never drank any alcohol except for Julian's Red Altar Wine - wine that was supposedly blessed at a discount liquor store in Paw-Paw, Michigan - a three-hour and forty-seven minute drive my mother often made from her driveway to the Julian Wine's graveled parking lot. She was a religious woman.

I repeated the offer but this time with less intoxicant volume. "Would you like to have a little something to drink, mom? Perhaps orange juice or water?"

"Oh no! I'm just fine but you can have a beer if you like."

Even the room was confused. The air could barely carry such blasphemous words. My mother hated beer. The taste made her nauseous, other people drinking beer made her nauseous and the smell made her nauseous. She would start her lecturing the second she heard the pop a cap makes when it is pried from its bottle.

“You wouldn’t mind if I had a beer?” My breath was short and unsure. Slowly I rose from the sofa and stood on the soles of my feet.

In walking to the fridge, I couldn't help but turn my head back several times starring at this little foreigner with the Einstein hair sitting on *my* mother's sofa - my grandmother's sofa. Everything in that room was waiting for something to happen.

I got the said beer out of the fridge and also a lemon. It was risky but I took the lemon, cut a wedged slice and hung it on to the rim of the bottle and carefully walked back to this stranger.

She tapped the sofa's cushion. "Come sit here."

I did.

"Closer. Move your behiney closer to me.”

I did.

“I am so glad you're here. How long are you staying?"

I peeled my dry lips apart creating an opening for an answer to work its way out into the room but my words were shoved back into my mouth by her unbreakable line of chatter.

"We have so much to do. First, we need to plant those flowers I bought. They're downstairs in the... the room downstairs… you know… in the three big bags. I bought some beautiful red begonias and yellow daisies and some tiny blue flowers with white eyes. They're the… I don't know what their name is."

Every year Violet would plant plastic flowers in her garden. And on every summer Tuesdays and Thursdays she would water her garden during the hours allowed by the water gods at City Hall. Watering her plastic begonias on the regulated days for my mother was patriotic. She thought it her civic duty.

"They're all downstairs in the... the room, you know, the room downstairs. Go get them for me."

I welcomed any reason to leave these four walls. I needed to clear her head, to walk on familiar ground. I had to make sure reality, as I know it, was somewhere waiting for me outside this room. The windows behind the sofa offered little corroborating evidence.

I was about to stand when my mother grabbed my hand and pulled me closer into the sofa.

"Sit back down. You can bring the flowers to me later."

I did.

"I bought them at Michaels. They had a huge sale a month of weeks ago and I bought two summer's worth of flowers..." Violet took a deep breath and continued in unstoppable excitement.

"Did Lil'Vi call me today? I can't remember. You know she calls me everyday. Rain or shine. Last week, yes

I think it was last week when I put that paper... uhh... the... you know, the... wax paper over my cabbage horns cause it was raining at the church. Do you know how to make the cabbage horns? For the life of me, I don't know why you don't learn how to make them or speak Slovak. What if I die? Who's going to make them for the church? Who's going to make them for the dead people's wakes when I not here? Well, I can't worry about me dying right now, I need to make a hundred plus thirty-two for the church's party. They need them in the morning for after Mass, the long Mass. Oh my God, is it THIS Sunday? Do you know when I gotta do that? Maybe Lil'Vi would remember the day. Yes, Lil'Vi will remember. We better call her now."

Violet looked under her purse and shuffled through stacks of papers topping the table in front of her looking for what she forgot.

"Not sure, but I do know that I told some man... What am I looking for?"

The little Einstein looked at me for some answer but I didn't have a clue what was happening. Leaves moved closer to the window, the sun winked again at my mother - a sun that was tired and getting ready to leave.

"Oh yes, I almost forgot. We need to get my driver's license *expanded.* You don't have to worry, I have the picture already, they just need to check my driving and expand the expiration numbers on my license. I already have it here somewhere in my purse."

"You mean renewed? Had it expired?"

Violet began empting her purse on the cluttered table.

"Mom, forget it for now. I believe you. Later. Look for it later."

"You know I've been driving since I was twelve. I will tell the man that. Maybe he can just stamp it and skip me driving all together. What do ya think?"

"I don't know, mom... I don't know."

"Remind me to bring him some candy."

Behind the chatter, snapshots of my mother played inside my head. Numerous pictures squeezed themselves together. I could see all of them at the same time. I saw something in my mother under the chatter. It is hard to explain but there was a peaceful clarity in her voice even though there was no order.

[That was about the time when
I learned to listen more closely...
without my ears.]

"Well, it could have been the pastor. I told someone that I would bring two trays of my cabbage horns. Everyone loves those horns. Maybe we should make some for Richard at the bank. After all, he is the president and he does print out all my music sheets without charging me a dime. He doesn't have to do that, you know. He really should be Jewish."

The tickertape of words, jammed into sentences fell out of my mother's mouth yet seamlessly sewn together.

"Wait. Wait a minute. Maybe it was that funny looking priest with the tight Toni permanent? You know who I'm talking about. I think he keeps the lotion on too long but I wouldn't say anything. I like him. He's kind. Did you notice his hair? It's so kinky. Sometimes it's like a Brillo pad and then after a week or two, if he washes it often, it turns wavy like Philomela's hair. But when he puts all they grease on it that's when it's turns more like Loretta's husband on 23rd and Kedzie. Remember Loretta?"

"Mom, isn't Loretta's husband bald?"

"Oh know. When did that happen? I got to send her a prayer card."

As my mother continued seaming her words into a line disconnected thoughts, I slipped off my shoes and sunk into the sofa, resting my head on the back cushion. The room was now yellowed by the tired sun; lace curtains moved closer into the conversation by the afternoon breeze; and the lemon pearls on the rim of my cold beer reclined in favor.

My mother hardly noticed that I had surrendered myself to her stories and the tiny breath that separated them. We were unplugged from the world. What I thought was real just minutes ago had lost its grip. I allowed myself to be cradled in the nonsensical, cockeyed rhythm of my mother's chatter. The crazy babbling and chopped up sentences were more engaging than trying to interpret their meaning.

In those moments, I was encouraged to pursue my mother's *flanerie*. I had to go with her. I had to go where she was. I knew I could always find my way back home.

< UNITED AIRLINES >
FLIGHT: #841 Tues Jan 17
DEPART: Chicago at 9:55 PM
ARRIVE: California at 3:57 PM
CANCELED
Rebook return February 28

STAGE TWO

SYMPTOMS

Difficulty doing routine tasks:
cooking, laundry, using the phone.
Problems recognizing sights and
sounds that used to be familiar.
Decreased capacity to pay bills.

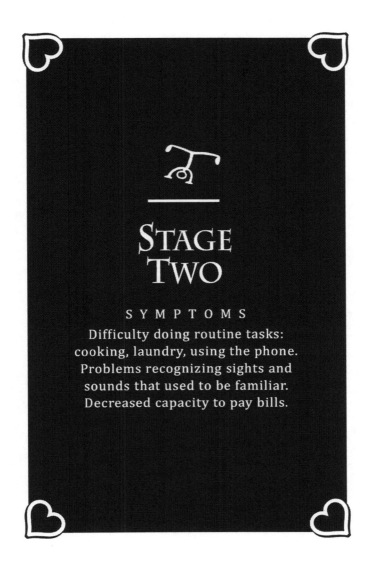

16.
CEMETERY PICNICS

"Where did that bag of breads go to, I lay it right here?"

"Look, girls, look for that bag. There will be no sandwiches, no picnic without bread."

With hardly a breath break, Violet had chopped her line of thought and had turned up her volume to maximum shrill, "Pavel. Pavel..." She had turned to her girls, "Where is your father? Suzka go look for your father. Ask him where he put the breads."

Violet whipped her hand in the air and had turned her body 180 to a group of tightly stuffed bags. One of them was hiding the breads.

[That summer in the 50's, the first
Corvette was built in Flint, Michigan
and the Chicago Cubs signed their

first black player Ernie Banks.
I still have his autographed picture
someplace.]

Violet had prepared and bagged all the food for the picnic in the back kitchen behind the store. The kitchen was one of four rooms where Violet and her husband lived and started their family. All morning Violet made sausages and sauerkraut, plum dumplings and blueberry bublania. She cut slices of meat stuck in clear jello and wrapped them carefully in brown paper; Pavel's favorite.

One by one she carried the bags with meats and tins filled with cookies to the front of the store, the showroom part which now was flooded with the sides for the day: blankets and pillows, sunbonnets and sweaters, bug spays, mosquito repellents and two bottles of Campho Phenique. Stacked haphazardly on a group of bellied bags near the door were four mismatched aluminum folding-chairs with worn crisscrossed webbing. The floor had lost its space. Violet carefully stacked everything she would forget. Every needed item for a family picnic and their duplicates waited at the store's door like an unruly line of kindergarteners seconds before a bell announced its recess.

Violet shuffled her way around the boxes and bags looking for what she forgot.

"Suzka, stop it. Stop jumping around. "Violet put a theatrical shiver of medical seriousness in her voice and placed her full hand over her chest. "I swear, you're gonna give me a nervous breakdown. Don't make me go crazy... you hear me?"

The six-year old child showed no concern over her mother's missing breads, "Mom, just ask Jesus to find the breads."

"Don't be sacrilegious. That's St. Anthony's job. Go, go, go. Look for your father. I'll talk to Anthony by myself. "Violet made the sign of the cross like she was scratching the breath of an itch. "Jesus Christ, give me strength."

Neighboring roaches had looked out from the walls at the bagged utopia but kept their distance. They lived next door at Polanski Pizza, a popular Polish family-owned establishment. The roaches ate pizza droppings of sausage and cheese and after they were fat and sleepy they would crawl punch-drunk through the walls to Violet and Pavel's side late into the night. Violet hated the drunken roaches. She would throw telephone books on them and ask the girls to jump on the books securing their demise. Pavel would clear the remains after Violet stopped screaming and his girls got bored jumping from book to book.

"Paaaavel! Where are you? It's already 10 o'clock. We're gonna be late." Violet's wristwatch and the store's clock read 8:32. It's not that she couldn't read time properly she simply manipulated and greatly exaggerated the numbers to her benefit.

It was going to be a hot Sunday, the first in a long line of the summer's family picnics. During the winter, every Sunday the family would go to the house of Violet's parents where everyone ate, laughed, talked over each other and loudly argued together. When the snow melted and the first wrapped tulip popped up from the hard soil, it was Pavel's turn. He would take his family to picnic on his parents' graves. Cemetery picnics were old bohemian traditions in Chicago. And the first Sunday of the summer was the most sacred. It was mandatory, demanding an appearance as any wake or marriage would.

Anything related to the church or death came with social obligations. Some events required compulsory appearances, which brought everyone in the family out into the open: out of sicknesses, hospital stays, probations or protective witness programs.

Violet walked outside and handed two cloth bags to Pavel. "These bags need to be in the front close to me; this one on the seat and this one on the floor between my legs. My legs will hold it tight from spilling." She wiped her hands on her apron and looked closely over the piled collection. She looked at her husband as if she were handing him an I.O.U. for future appreciation. There was no time to waste. No time for expressing the slightest sign of gratitude. She hurried herself back into the store.

A cup of steaming coffee sat on the car's roof. It was early. The sun was young and unaware of its strength. Pavel slid back his hat and scratched his head at the pile of bags gathered on the sidewalk. Suzka sat on the curb resting her thoughts on her knees and hiding from her mother.

"What's that old man across the street lookin' at?" the girl asked her father.

Pavel looked up. A man who adequately filled a folding chair like a bohemian Buddha had focused his attentions on Pavel's car packing from across the street. His tongue and lips worked in unison rolling a wet fat cigar from one side of his mouth to the other. Navy blue pants mooned over his large belly. Under his belly two legs spread out like wings of a stuffed turkey but with white socks and brown slippers.

Pavel waved.

The old man couldn't see Pavel's neighborly gesture or he simply refused to respond. His eyes were flattened behind a thick dark glass framed in horn rims. His head never moved, a standoff of sights. The old man kept his wave to himself but offered a reprehensible opinion that walked across the street by itself to Pavel – '*your'a doy'ng id all wrong*'.

Pavel stared back thinking, '*Whatcha lookin' at ole man?*'

On weekdays a jumbled pile of cars parked by Europeans who spoke bad *parking* would have blocked the view and muffled his remarks from crossing the street, but this was Sunday. Parking customers were at home. Family businesses were closed.

Pavel adjusted his hat and returned to packing the bags in the car. He recommitted himself to the day.

Their store was one in a row of storefronts. A jumbled collection of family businesses started fathers-and-mothers ago when dreams were only dreams and families were bigger than bad luck. The storefronts were long and tightly lined next to each other on a busy street. Only a thin slice of air separated them, the slice of space where the day took a rest from the heat of the sun. All the buildings were the same: store showrooms in the front, living spaces in the back and separate apartments on its second floor. We lived behind the store in four rooms.

The front face was the only thing visible from the street; a face that did not match the rest of its flat brick body. On both ends were two large windows where neon tubes hung. The glass tubes illuminated a humming blue color outside its casing and twisted to spelling the store's name – *VIP Dry Cleaners.* On the window's inside floor was a line of potted cattails.

People on the street looked over the cattails to see Violet working at the counter. Kids and Imogene could not see Violet. They would have to believe she was somewhere behind the windowed glass.

[Imogene was a little person
who lived in one of the apartments
above the cleaning store.]

When local customers walked into the store with their soiled cloths to be cleaned and mended, a bell loosely fastened to a metal strip at the top of the door, wiggled. The sound like a nervous giddy schoolgirl talking to her friends about her first kiss, could be heard in the kitchen forty feet away. The bell called on Violet to come quickly to the front of the store, a customer was waiting.

Before the clothing went to the commercial cleaning factory, alterations were made in the back of the store's showroom: a sewing area with three long folding tables.

The center table had one Singer sewing machine. On Each side were piles of suits, pants and dresses waiting for repairs. There were threads, a number of scissors, some with pinking edges and wax chalk markers. And buttons, buttons everywhere, some packaged and labeled with the garments name, others lost and alone. The floor was covered with short threads. They were disabled casualties, the runaways of the cleaning store business, lying dead on the battleground after the alterations. Violet would gather all of them together and bury them once a week in the Hoover.

When the mending was complete and the garments were returned from the factory after being chemically cleaned, Violet would place them carefully on a paper covered wire hanger with fancy cursive lettering - *VIP Cleaners*. Pavel would deliver them to the garments' homes when he was not working at Western Electric.

Next to the cleaning store was Polanski Pizza and next to the pizza store was a tavern with dark floors and poor lighting. When Violet couldn't find her husband, she would tell Suzka to go to the tavern and look for her father. Violet hated Pavel's drinking. She hated the taste of whiskey and the smell of beer.

[The world's most famous taste
in beer at that time was Schlitz.
The beer that made Milwaukee famous.]

"What's that smell? It smells like sewer gas." She would squish her face and move the faint smell with a waving hand for the dramatic effect and then argue with Pavel for hours.

Violet would whisper to her girls, "Your father's drunkenness is the cross we have to bear. Remember Marie's husband Ralph? He was a terrible drunkard. Remember at Stella's wedding, when he fell over two tables, drunk, stinking drunk? He lay there on his belly, on broken glass in a pool of whiskey. His daughter, who was about your age, went over to her pitiful father and picked him up and took him to their car. And now she's a doctor. She took that cross she had to bear and got a degree in medicine."

"Go down to the tavern and look for your father. He'll come if you go get'em. Tell him I have dinner on the table and it's getting cold. Tell him you're hungry, no... tell him you're starving. Act weak, but don't go into faintin'. God only knows what's on that bar room's floor. Tell him to hurry."

Suzka walked in the tavern and stopped at its entrance. Her eyes were closed inside to the new darkness. She brought in the light behind her to back her up. No one could see the little girl, but a cockeyed pigtail silhouette gave her away. She was shorter than half the room. The top half was where all the drinking and talking took place. After her inside eyes opened, she walked past a long line of bar stools, touching each one as she passed them, except for the stools that had butts pressed into them. Suzka knew the face of her father's butt.

When she got to her father, she would squeeze between the stools and tug at his leg to get his attention.

"Mom wants you to come home right now. She has dinner on the table."

The other butts in the tavern knew Suzka. They would laugh and say, "Little one, tell your mother your father will be there shortly. He's helping me move an electric icebox for the poor old widowed lady upstairs... Would you like a pickle?"

"No Sir, my mom has dinner waiting. I could take some pretzels though. That shouldn't ruin my dinner."

But today is Sunday and the tavern is closed for business. The owner and its loyal customers are packing their own cars with sausages and Old Crow for the summer's first picnic.

Violet balanced two wax-papered trays on her hipbone and side shuffled her body through the store's maze that led her outside.

"Pavel, why is all this stuff still sitting out here? What have you been doing? How are you going to get everything packed inside the car? We're not gonna get a parking place near the grave unless we leave in the next five minutes. You know how crowded the cemetery gets." Half of Violet's words bent with her body into the station wagon as she continued talking and fussing.

"Put those trays right here. This one goes on top of everything. But not so on the top that the heat goes to it. Put it on top as not to get smashed. And this one..." Her words were ahead of her thoughts with no place to go.

Violet stood outside the car in the sea of bags and looked over the situation like the captain of the Titanic. Her five-foot aproned body faced her husband holding two more cloth bags in his arms. Pavel hadn't moved. His full mind was under the driver's seat of the station wagon where he securely wrapped and placed his bottle of Old Crow whiskey.

"And put those flowers in last. They go on top of everything else." ...flowers that Violet will plant on the graves of her in-laws.

With conclusive vibrancy, Violet's tone changed. She spoke as if she was reading the last line in a long novel. "Ok, that's it. We're ready. Let's go. I'll get my purse."

In less than five minutes, Mira, Suzka, Lil'Vi and Pavel jammed everything into the station wagon with no order.

Their picnic was stacked to the car's ceiling looking like sausage meats stuffed in its casing. Lil'Vi sat on her mother's lap in the front. Suzka and her sister Mira sat in the back; the last two pieces in the summer Sunday's puzzle.

"*You are my sunshine, my only sunshine, you make me happy when skies are blue. You'll never know dear how much I love you. Please don't take my sunshine away...* Did you lock the store door..." a question heard but never stood a chance of being answered.

"Turn around, Pavel. Go back. I'll jump out and double check its lock."

*

The cemetery where Grandma Agnes and Grandpa Otis lived was not far. They were buried in Chicago's west side where a large population of dead people resided. The most notable residents included Sam Battaglia, Anthony Acardo and Al Capone. Pavel told his girls their ghosts made the cemetery a safe place to rest.

In a short time they reached the tall iron gates. Suzka's eyes worked intently outside her sockets. She was concentrating harder than her years were used to looking for the tall cement angel with open arms and blank eyes. The angel was close to where they would have their picnic. Everyone Suzka did not know lived there. They were family.

A newly tarred road curved and wandered through the headstone'd community. Cars driving in the opposite direction would often have to roll over the mowed grass and buried bones of relatives living on the edges.

Everyone laid close together, some on top of another. Their spot was planned and withstood the wars inside the family. Cemetery plots were purchased years before there were dreams of weddings. Stonemasons would add the chiseled name into the family's marble headstone the day a nervous man brought a box of candy to an old lady with a beautiful daughter. But even with assurance set in stone, final burials were tenuous and were often negotiated, gambled and argued over.

All Suzka knew was every summer Sunday she would go with her family to have a picnic on the bones of Agnes and Otis. Their porcelain faces were glued to a marble stone where any five-year old could securely set her juice glass.

The cemetery was the place where children chased each other without reason, old men smoked fat cigars and drank whiskey in hard plastic juice glasses and mothers blanketed the graves with delicious meats and breads. This was the place where the little Suzka's family would have their picnics and her father would be happy.

"There's a place to park, it's close to Otis and Agnes. Hurry Pavel, before someone takes that spot."

Pavel's foot was in heavy sleep on the brake pedal. His arm rested itself over the window ledge. It was already a hot day. The smell of lilacs and sausage was thick and moved slow with the traffic. Pavel's face was calm in thought and gave every sign of not listening to a word Violet was saying. Today he would eat sandwiches, drink beer and rest in his youth in the arms of his past.

Pavel missed his mother. Every year he would cry with Old Crow on the anniversary of her death. Violet never met Agnes or Otis. She only visits them at picnics and talks of them in arguments with Pavel. Pavel never liked that. He would leave and visit Old Crow or Jack Daniels, whoever was home at the time.

"Is that Gladys over there?" Violet waves her full hand over Pavel's nose to a woman resembling a Gladys. "She didn't wave back. I wonder why she ignored me." Violet squints and continues her wave but with less enthusiasm. "Maybe that wasn't her after all."

Gladys's ignored wave would be the first in a number of waves lost in the cemetery, waves looking for some recognition.

All the cars moved slowly, bumper to bumper with arms and heads popping out at their sides. They ribboned the pathways and eventually parked themselves. Doors opened into the street for old fat ladies with cotton black dresses and big breasts and big hats to be pulled out of the car's back seat by the men who married their daughters. Trunk lids opened their mouths filled with their picnics.

Pavel carefully opened the back door of his station wagon preventing any anxious bags from running out.

"Be careful with those begonias. Give those two bags to Suzka." Lil'Vi stood under the transactions with her arms extended out.

"And give those baby flowers to Lil'Vi." The fresh flowers will be planted above the skulled bones of grandparents no one ever met. In the winter Violet would plant plastic flowers. Their petals could hold the snow with no deadly consequences.

Otis and Agnes died when Pavel was young. His mother died of pleurisy, a few months later his father died of *the drink*. In their own time, they laid stiff in a wood box balanced on two chairs in their living room. Agnes wore a Sunday summer cotton dress and a ribbon in her hair. Flowers brought from neighbors' gardens and placed in chipped glass vases tried to dress the odor in the summer's hot room. Otis wore a dusty wool suit with a preserving smell and mismatched buttons. It was cold that winter. Neighbors brought pine branches and holly in the familiar chipped vases. All flowers died months ago.

"Pavel, be careful, watch them girls so they don't walk on the heads of those people's graves."

Suzka's older sister Mira carried the blanket and two aluminum-folding chairs to the grave for the older visitors who wanted to pay their respects, eat pickles and sip Old Crow in lemonade glasses They would talk about their bladders and bowels and about who died and had biggest attended funerals in the past year.

[James Dean died that year, but
he wasn't buried at our cemetery.]

"Girls, girls, quit clownin' around and help me. Where's Suzka? That girl's gonna be the death of me... where'd she go?"

Violet laid out the blanket over the bumpy-grassed bones of Pavel's mother and father.

"Anyone know where Suzka went?"

Suzka was always missing. When no one was looking, she would run away and disappear behind the headstones with carved names she could not read and gravediggers could not pronounce. Jumping from stone to stone, staying out of sight. She was audacious but also cemetery savvy and quite familiar with the residents' unspoken rules – you don't jump or walk up the bones below. It was a known fact that the graved ghosts could grab the running feet of little girls and pull them into the dirt, if they had a mind to. Stone angels with blank eyes and no pupils could only watch. It can be scary for the unadventurous. Some headstones were flat to the ground. The bones below pulled their stones down with them just to confuse everyone and make room for the littlest visitors to do their cartwheels.

Suzka made her way back to the grave for a quick salami sandwich. Pavel was lying on the picnic blanket dreaming. His one arm was around Lil'Vi. Mira was resting her back against a neighboring headstone while reading *Diary of Anne Frank.*

Violet caught Suzka in her eye. “Where have you been girl? And look at those legs of yours. How did those feet of yours get that dirty so quickly. Good Lord girl, you’re gonna drive me to an early grave.”

Violet extended a bucket out with one hand and pointed to a water spigot standing three feet out from the ground. “Go now and fill this with water." The spigot leaned slightly to one side and had a drippy mouth. “We need the water for plantin’. Go. Go ahead now.”

Sweat dripped down Suzka's pigtails. It was sticky hot. If she touched the air she would leave her print. The afternoon's heat jellied everything in its place. Violet wore a large straw hat that protected her from the sun but not from the heat. "Where are your shoes Suzka?"

"I donno."

Brassy sounds from horns and tambourines distracted their attention. Thick air muffled its clatter but its intent was clear.

Suzka squinted her eyes toward the music. There was a change in her face.

"It's time. It's time. The parade is starting. I gotta go, mom, I gotta go." Suzka jumped in her body and nervously wiggled herself with intentions. “I gotta go, I gotta go."

"Ok, ok. Don’t act all crazy now. Go ahead but be careful and don’t walk on anybody’s bones."

Suzka ran toward the music as fast as she could between the stone markers and the cemented angels. She ran fast and hard avoiding the tarred road that was hot like nothing else under her feet. In her run she saw at a distance the statue of the Virgin Mary with open arms. The virgin’s head swayed back and forth above the crowd. The statue was carried in a wood basket and elevated in the air by six men wearing fedoras and porkpie hats.

Breathless from running Suzka ran to the tree she knew she could climb for a better look. This year the climb will be easier. The tree got smaller or she was bigger.

Behind the Virgin statue was an elaborately dressed man wearing a silk robe jeweled in gold appliqués. He wore a tall satiny hat that made him look much taller than he actually was. The hat matched his sequined shoes. The fancy man spread open his arms and sprinkled the crowd with blessed water from a silver rattle. Men wearing white choir dresses over red cassocks surrounded him. They carried the clouds of smoke.

The roadway was lined with a hundred parade-ians flanked with banners, fans, tall candles and long poles with silver crosses on the top. Plum feathered guards with brassy instruments played the music. The heavy air from trombones and other wind instruments solemnly dragged their sounds. All the children waved their hands in front of their eyes as though they were slapping flies.

On the sidelines, standing over the edged graves, old women hunched over their rosaries. They counted their beads on their lips. Young fathers ran with the parade moving closer to the virgin statue in order to pin dollar bills to the virgin's cloak.

Cheers usually heard at other parades had been replaced with chanting and songs about virgins and queens, wretches and temptations. All the children jumped up and down with their mouths wide open and their tongues pushed out in hopes of catching a few drops of the blessed water that was sprinkled in the air by the sequined man. Everyone was solemnly excited and had joined the parade to its end. Ground ants and summer beetles from the tasty graves were the last to follow behind.

The procession had ended at the stone grotto for the high mass. Suzka never stayed much past the parade. She believed there was no good reason for anyone under the years of five to continue. The little explorer walked back to Agnes and Otis for the glass of lemonade she left on the ledge of their headstone.

17.
OTHER PLOTS

[This summer Queen Elizabeth was a
TV movie series, the Chevrolet Corvette
was built in Bowling Green, Kentucky

and the Chicago Cubs came in 4th place
in the NL Central. Ernie Banks was 74.
I still have that autographed picture
some place.]

My mother leaned over the railing on the second floor. "I'm leaving now Suzka. Are you ready? I'm going to get the car out of the garage. You meet me in the front quickly and then I'll take you to your *Starbuckies* for coffee. Hurry. Don't lollygag."

I was still lying on the couch under the warm covers, my butt stuck to its leather, one leg hung over the backrest. The thoughts of winged stone angels, picnic sandwiches and parades left my head. Life was easier when blessings were sprinkled in the air and absolutions were handed out like party favors with penances freely given for everything nasty. Ribbons of Latin circled our faith with its illusions and delusions, its mysteries and aha moments of glory. No one puts on a show like the Catholics.

Violet yelled out her final warning "Hurry now. I got my coat on and I'm leaving."

The garage door closed. I jumped off the couch and flew into my routine. Pee, brush, blush, pull up my tights and slip on a t-top; then pull back my hair and claw-clip everything to the top of my head. It would take my mother about eight minutes from the slam of the back door to the car's first honk in front of the house. I could get out the door in seven.

I grabbed my red sling-back heels as I ran up the steps and in seconds slam locked the door behind me.

"I'm ready... let's go." The words fell out of a yawn.

Mom always looked amazed. Her kooky looking artist daughter didn't look half bad but she didn't have the time to spend acknowledging her approval. Mother was in a hurry to get to the place outside of herself. I would lipstick myself after '*Starbuckies*'. And off we drove quickly, barely stopping at the corner's stop sign.

"Suzka, are you sure the door is locked? I'm gonna turn around and you jump out and double check it's locked." The cement curb didn't get a chance to move aside.

Before the car could officially stop, she spoke. "Now go... go hurry out and check the door then we'll go to your '*Starbuckies*'. Some things never change.

"Are you excited about going to the cemetery?"

"Yea mom, I'm excited. I'm thrilled to death." I was still in sleep and slowly sipping the thoughts of coffee.

"Don't talk of death like that."

The car was warm; the early warmth only a young sun can bring into a car.

She kept talking but I heard very little. There was some kind of mumbling and then a yawning silence met us half way.

*

It took only 15 minutes to get to the cemetery. Violet understood traffic lights. That was good. She just didn't pay mush attention to them. Graved relatives were waiting for her.

The large virgin queen with open arms met us at the entrance. The granite queen could be seen for miles. On each side were twelve-foot high cast-iron gates with patterns of loops and twists and gold leafing. At night the gates closed the cemetery. Violet turned into the entrance without much assistance from the car's brakes. The gates leaned to one side making room for her wide turn.

The tarred road squirmed its way through the thousands of headstones that popped out of the ground in no proper order. The older stones leaned tiredly to one side. Specks of color surfaced here and there from fresh wreaths and small plants. They rested on wire arms with their mouths opened to the sun. The older oaks reduced down in diminishing numbers to where the newer graves were planted. There was a warm familiarity about it all.

Stone angels with visionless eyes and large tufted wings dominated the grounds. Their plastered hands reached down in blessing. A few of the smaller angels sat on tops of grave markers with their legs crossed and with their heads held in their hands. But it was the virgins and saints that stood on pillars who watched the goings-on with holiness.

Scattered in between the sainted markers were lawn crypts; tiny stone houses with gold doors locked and unfurnished inside. Behind the doors whole families slept forever in one tiny room.

Cemeteries are homes for spectacular creatures of legends. They feed the earth during the day and at night they dress themselves in leaves and dance in the moon's light. When the moon is finished the dead simply lie down, pull the earth over their bones and gaze at the remaining stars. Restless souls who could not sleep during the night often pass by the daytime visitors like a whiff of rich air with the smells of honeysuckle and decay.

We passed Agnes and Otis without stopping. My mother offered a quick wave not expecting one in return and not turning her head for a second to catch the illusion of their acknowledgement.

She lifted her hand off the steering wheel to push her sunglasses closer up to the bifocals underneath. The car swerved. "What's down there?" The car veered again in the direction of her pointed finger.

"Graves, mom. Just more and more graves."

The car stopped for a brief moment. A pigeon sitting on cement cross looked around for a cool place to nap, perhaps in the soffit of an angel's wing. The feathered creature looked like he recognized my mother.

"Look, over there. Do you see that procession?" Pause. "Auh, someone's gonna be buried today." Violet's hand ran the *sign-of-the-cross* across her face without the slightest thought of its religious intent. "It looks like he's important. Not politician important mind you... there's not enough cars for that." She took her foot off the brake and continued driving.

"You count the cars Suzka. I can't. I'm driving."

A crunch and then a heavy thumping scraped the bottom of the car.

"Watch the road mom." I felt the sound through my feet. I twisted my neck far back over my shoulder and looked out the window. A blizzard of tiny white, lavender and red flower petals flew around in the air.

"I think you rolled over a grave mom and one of those flowered wreaths."

"Don't be silly." She attempted to look out her window at a side mirror but the mirror was in no condition to show her the damages she left behind. It was hanging off the car by a glob of wires and torn duct tape, remnants from a tollbooth incident. The booth slammed into my mother's car the summer before I moved in with her.

"Just sit back and relax. I've been driving since I was twelve."

I dare not say anything. I was just grateful that everyone she ran over was already dead.

The cemented angels prayed for their safety.

"Do you see your father anywhere?" She turned her head and stared at me, asking in a strange voice. "He's around here someplace."

I put my coffee in the holder and looked around. "I thought you knew where he was mom."

"I do... but they moved everybody around. I hate it when they move every… one… around." It was as if her memory got dizzy and fell out of her head.

The car stopped.

My mother stared at the windshield. Her eyes squinted into the sunlight trying to remember. She moved her head from side to side squishing everything in front of her together, trying to make sense of it all. Her face was distorted as if it was turned inside out in a desperate appeal to the gods inside her. There weren't any road signs and even if there were, it wouldn't have made a difference. She still wouldn't know.

"Mom... Mom."

Her eyes were blank, filled with blindness like the stone angels. Sweat water covered the steering wheel. Outside the air wrinkled in its own heat. The lilacs marinated the sky into purple.

"Mom. Mom are you ok?"

We sat there quietly - the cemetery's skyline in front of us with its abrupt stoned figures and structures, black and gray. Thousands of angels looked at us waiting for something to happen.

Her fists dug into the steering wheel - she barely moved a muscle in fear of being exposed. Buttons of water sat on her forehead. Violet closed her eyes inhaling a time she couldn't remember. She only had her heart and her wit to call on.

I couldn't stand the silence but my tongue had turned to stone. A ground's attendant had walked by. He paused at first and then glanced at us with assumed indifference. He lowered his head and used one hand as a sun visor and pressed it against the glass. He tapped on the window gently and asked, "You ok in there?"

My mother fixated her eyes on the man nose-close at her window and focused her entire brain as best she could. When nothing registered, she yelled at me "What does he want? Does he want a ride? You're not picking up any hitchhikers are you? He's gonna kill us. You know he's gonna rob us first and then kill us."

"No, no, no mom. He's fine. He must work here."

"Lock your door. Lock all the doors."

I leaned over my mother and extended an *everything-is-ok* wave to the kindly man. The windows sealed us in tight. My mother was soundless. Outside a water spigot poked out from the ground. It leaned to one side dripping quietly onto the grass like a whisper in a sleeping baby's room.

"Where are we... where are we going?" Her words were slow creeping up from her throat where they broke and were cut in two.

"To see father. We're going to see father's gravesite, mom. Isn't that what you wanted to do?"

"I need to ask you a favor but you must promise?"

"Promise what mom? What do you want?"

"No, you have to promise."

"Ok. What is it?"

"I don't want to be here." Her promise got lost somewhere in its direction. "I want to go home. I want you to take me to my house but don't tell anyone."

"Ok. No problem. We can go now if you want to."

A car from behind blew its horn.

My heart jumped like a bird. And it was as if Lazarus himself slapped my mother in the face bringing her back to her senses. Her mind turned the corner.

"There it is! There they are! I can see it. Clear as it can be. Can you see it? You're father is right over there."

Her pointing finger hit my nose and nearly sliced it off my face. She had such a look about her that I almost burst out laughing. She broke into giddy laughter, stretching her throat sweetly and shaking her head. She put her hands together. "Your wicked father is gonna drive me crazy." There was youth in her bones.

Her sparked memory drove us to a neighboring section with some familiarity. She rolled the car over a buried curb and parked on the graved bones of some other poor soul.

"Come on, hurry, let's go. Get out of the car so I can lock it."

My interest in following lagged a couple of yards behind her pace. The smell of lilacs and fresh grass clippings comforted my nerves.

"Come on, come on. You don't want to get lost around here" – her words followed behind as if they were brain-crumbs for me to follow.

"I'm right behind you."

Cemetery plots were considered real estate to my mother's kind. Years ago, after the Depression, it was the tiny piece of land one could afford to buy, to stand on claiming it as their holding. A plot five feet by ten feet, barely a spec of an acre made them property owners.

They felt connected to the earth and securely grounded in ownership.

My mother had no intentions of being buried in the ground. I often thought this brave-looking woman was in reality scared out of her wits not necessarily of dying but of being buried in the ground. Maybe secretly she thought of all the bugs she killed, the roaches she brutally smashed to death under the weight of those torpedoing telephone books at a time when she was a young mother living in the cleaning store; perhaps she thought the entire roach community would crawl to her grave for revenge and finish her off, gorging themselves on her flesh. For whatever reason, my mother had other plans and made them known to me and to my sisters.

"I want to be laid in a polished silver casket with angel's heads at each corner and silver plated handles. My wake will need to be two days with a lot of finger food. Make sure to put two huge lush flower baskets on each side about yea tall (the yea tall measured about four inches above her standing position). And one of those big wreaths should have roses and calla lilies with the gold *Mother* ribbon crossing the wreath. You know, like those ribbons they use at the Miss America pageants. Lay that one on the top, over my legs. Tell the choir to sing the Our Father, Amazing Grace and Ave Maria."

She continued with hardly a space for a tiny breath, "And the procession of cars. Suzka you make sure you count them. There should be many. You would make your mother very happy if you can make sure there are fifty-eight, at least fifty-eight. I'd be happy with one more than fifty-eight but I'm not greedy. Greedy is a sin. After the Mass is all done with and I'm put in the crypt, then you can take everybody to Crystals for lunch. You pay."

I heard it a million times.

*

"Come on, come on now."

"I'm right behind you. I'm right behind you."

We walked to a marble-faced structure about the size of eight caskets high and sixteen across. The marble faced wall was cut in squares. Behind each square were bones in metal boxes decaying by themselves feeding no one. My father's bones were behind one of those squares.

We stood side-by-side in front of a marbled wall looking for the square with my father's nameplate glued in the center. I waited and watched while my mother made these brisk elongated movements, tapping on the marble squares while counting in fallen whispers. When she was confident in her resolve, she announced with graciousness and splendor, "Here it is."

Her arms fully opened like the stone angel at the main entrance. She stepped back and took a deep breath of the fresh morning air and said, "This is my surprise."

My face followed her.

"What do you think?" She asked.

I watched her carefully, my face nervously frowning for no particular reason.

"I bought all these slots in this section. Not just the two where your father and myself will be staying. I bought all these... ten in all." She made it sound like she made reservations at a Hilton, a family timeshare in the Caribbean Islands.

Then she came at me again as clean as a comet with wings bigger than the biggest in all the heavens. "You and your sisters and all your husbands... we'll all be together. You don't have to worry about where you're going. You'll be here."

What... what did she say?

"Suzka, pay attention. Did you hear me? Look. There are exactly ten slots here. Your father is in this one, rest his soul." Violet kissed her fingers and transferred her kiss onto the cold marble marked with my father's name.

"Now listen carefully 'cause after I die I don't want you and your sisters to be fighting over who gets which one."

Fighting... what did she say... oh we'll be fighting... I was flabbergasted.

"I'm gonna lay here, right next to your father. Now all these others are for you girls and your husbands."

The hairs on my body rose.

"Mom, what are you talking about? When did you do this?"

"Years ago. It was hard to keep this secret from you girls but I did. Now pay attention. This one is for Mira and this one for her husband. Lil'Vi will be here and her husband right next to her. Now over here on this side is where you will go. You're on the end. You can lay right here..."

For eternity? My eternity? *Oh my god, what in the hell did she do?*

"Who's this?" It appeared my mother's full plan was interrupted. Her voice changed and got rather serious. "Someone new moved in the next slot - the one next to you. No one told me about this."

My mother squished her nose to raise her bifocals as she leaned over to read the letters on the neighboring marbled square. The letters read Joseph DeGregario. She slowly whispered his name. "Joseph DeGregario." Then she paused for a long time. Obviously she was rearranging her original plan. All at once she looked at me, quite angelically and said, "It's a sign."

The rest of her body was stone-stuck. Her eyes moved back to Joseph. She was heavy in thought calculating the facts before her. "Look Suzka. All these people around him have different names. He has no one laying next to his name."

Her brains stopped thinking and surrendered to the gift given to her. "It's a sign for sure, a sign from God." My mother appeared to be in shock as if she saw the Virgin Mary herself.

"Look. Look right here. There is no place for a wife layin' next to him. He's not married. Joseph DeGregario is single."

Oh God make her stop.

She looked up to the skies. "Thank you Jesus and all the saints in heaven."

Violet checked the birth and death dates under his name. She didn't need to do the math. She had that look. She could die now. The sky's opened, the trees clapped, a breeze brought the sweet smell of wedding jasmine and lilacs.

"He's perfect and just a few years older than you."

Violet made the sign of the cross three times thanking everyone; God, Jesus, the virgins and all the saints she knew. "DeGregario. That's such a nice name. A nice Italian man."

The decision was consummated.

"You will be buried here, by Joseph. Yes, you will be right here... next to Joe. God wants that to be."

I stood staring at her for a moment with an unwilling delight at the grotesque charm of the moment around me. My mother mumbled her good fortune to the trees and the birds as we walked back to the car never looking back.

"Don't forget, we got to go and get my driver's license *expanded.* Then after that you can go and do whatever you do. For now, let's go to Crystals and have lunch."

"Mom, why don't I drive?"

She turned around and looked at me from head to toe.

"Why? You don't think I can drive? Don't be silly. I've been driving since I was twelve."

Pause.

"Just look at your feet. Is that paint on your sandals?"

[I looked down at my feet
the same way I did when I was little.
They looked like the shoes of an explorer.

My sandals were artistically covered
with the remains of an inspiration.]

18.
THE FLYING COMETS

"Just look at your feet! Mira's feet are not as dirty as your feet. Look. Look how nice and clean she is. You don't see her feet dirty do you?"

[That was a Sunday. Two days later the
Coronation of Queen Elizabeth II was televised
- the day that kick-started our love of television.
We owned a 16inch picture tube Magnavox.]

"I have no time to scrub you clean right now. I have all this stuff to put away from our picnic. The food, the breads, the jello..." When she was done with her list, she took one more look. "Good Lord, dirt does love you child."

Cemeteries, no matter how groomed and friendly they are, had dirt that wanted to leave. They would attach themselves to little girls who jump, run and cartwheel on the residents. Dirt would stick itself to bare feet and hide under the nail parts and in toe jams undetected. My father had to wash and scrub them away on those picnic nights and other nights when my mother worked late sewing buttons on customers' wedding clothes and funeral suits.

"Pavel. Pavel!" flew out of her as if her mouth was on fire. She looked down at me pitiful like and said, "Go. Go to your father and have him clean you up before you go to bed… Pavel!"

*

I had stood in the porcelain kitchen sink filled with warm water. The end of my legs disappeared under a cloud of bubbles. My father hated long back-bending baths in a tub so he replaced them with footbaths in the kitchen sink. He would tell me, "Dirt is like ketchup. At the end of the day, it all settles to the bottom."

My mom was busy making alterations on suits that customers brought into the cleaning store. She was normally finished before dinner, but on this day, a big weekend wedding and two funerals kept her busier than usual. Old clothes needed to be cleaned and pant cuffs hemmed for the big events. My father would have to bathe us girls and put us in our pajamas on those nights.

I loved sink baths. It was better for story telling. Plus the sink only had room for one set of feet. It was more private. My sink bath took the longest. My feet were dirtier than my sisters, dirt that only alley archeologists would collect from their digs.

I rested one arm on my father's shoulder for support and the other on the window frame above the sink. Outside the window I could see whether Stacy was in her yard. The window gave me a perfect view. Stacy's yard was in the front of her house. There was no grass. It was filled with undernourished dirt in unplanned piles and mounds. Wood planks led visiting guests from the street gate to their front door. When it rained the dirt turned to mud and stuck to Stacy's shoes. Her mom would yell all the time at Stacy and her brothers for tracking mud pies in the house. I could hear her in our kitchen.

On hot summer days the window brought in smells of dead fish. Buckets of smelt caught by Stacey's father that morning or the day prior were kept outside. When the sun was done his sons would dig a hole and build a pit for their cooking. At nighttime the fire would turn the boys' dark faces gold and their teeth into pearls. Music tickled everyone's feet. Dirt danced in circles. Laughing, singing and the deathless sounds of children carried on in the late summer night's heat and kept us awake. Under the covers, inside my head, I giggled and cartwheeled around the fire with Stacy until I fell asleep.

"Com'on Papa, tell me the story again about the flies."

It was awkward for me to call my father 'papa.' I thought *papa* but said *father.* Everyone in the house called him father. *Wait 'til your father comes home young lady;* or *Ask your father;* or *Go check if your father's drinking.* Father washed my feet in the kitchen sink - Papa told me the stories like the one about the Performing Fly Comets.

"Don't you want to hear a different story? Suzka, you know the whole story by heart, nearly word for word." He took a deep breath of resolve. "When I get too old to tell it, you better be the one to tell it to me."

In reality, I knew it was my father's favorite.

"It's just the best story ever. Com'on Papa... and no shortcuts. I want to hear everything from the beginning to the end. Don't leave anything out. Now that I'm five, I know more when you skip stuff."

"What about the magic banana story?"

"That's not a story, that's a magic trick, which I haven't figured out yet. I'm gonna talk to Stacey about that. She knows just about everything. She'll be able to figure it out."

"Stacy huh... How could I forget?"

I put my nose to the window to see if Stacy was in her yard. "You know, she is quite now-ledged, especially about magic tricks. Gypsies know just about everything there is to know about magic."

Stacy was exactly my same size. We were both explorers and secret friends. Stacy had black shiny long hair that separated over her dark shoulders and a canopy of bangs shading her black almond eyes. Her mother told her she looked like her grandmother when she was about Stacy's age living in a small town in Turkey. Stacy's grandmother is dead now.

A wire fence with large square openings, large enough for small hands to squeeze through, separated us. The fence made it easy to share secrets and licorice. Near the bottom of the fence was a wood ledge that we would step on and reach over when we needed to exchange bigger secrets and uncut sandwiches.

My friend Stacy had four brothers. She was the youngest and the only girl. They all had black hair, shorter than Stacy's but longer than most boys I knew.

They smoked cigarettes. There was always a white cigarette tucked behind the boys' dark ears. They were scary cool to most people. I loved scary cool.

When our bird died, a canary and yellow in color, my father buried the lifeless creature in the corner of our tiny yard close to the fence. Stacy reverently watched from the other side, standing tall and soldier straight. I saw Stacy's right hand cover her heart through the whole burial. She saluted at the end when my father tapped down the mud pile with his shovel. Stacy was my best friend.

"You better not tell your mother about Stacy. She's doesn't like their wild ways. It's best she stays on her side of the fence and you stay on our side. That way there's no trouble. And don't let your mother catch you even thinkin' about going over to Stacy's yard through the alleyway."

My father added more soap on the soiled washcloth. He looked down into the sink where the clouds of bubbles were slowly drowning in a pool of dark gray water. The sink's sides were edged scummy-like in alley dirt.

"Sometimes I think you are dead set on making your mother crazy."

"What you lookin' at in the bubbles for? Com'on now, tell me the story about your workin' in the factory with the flies."

During the week my father worked at Western Electric in Cicero. A huge factory with a whistle that was heard for miles telling all the workers it was time to come to work. He worked long hours. My sisters and I were fast asleep when he finished his workday. He would peek in our room and glance for a moment at our closed faces. My face was never really closed. I pretended to sleep.

"Common' now. We don't have all night papa."

"Ok. Now let me see... It was a warmer day than usual. Winter was at the end of its cold. The bus let me off at the work stop. Leo was with me. Now normally the bus fumes fill my nose on both sides but this day a tiny bit of jasmine snuck in and tickled my hairs telling me it was spring. Leo and I walked into the factory and took the elevator going up to our department. The minute those elevator doors opened, I knew it was goin' to be a good flying day. All the windows were cracked wide open. Fresh city air filled the room."

"All us guys walked through the maze of maybe a hundred work tables and machines. Mine was in the back close to a line of opened windows. I just got settled and then it started. They saw me. That's when they all came rushin' over to my station, buzzin' around my work head. They kept buzzin' all morning long. Flies. Big flies; flies that spent all winter just getting' fat. They would do circles and dives, showing off with all kinds of flying maneuvers just to get my attention. A few sat on my tools walking back and forth showing their muscles. Did you know that flies have muscles?"

I didn't know that.

My father continued with his personal analogy. "You know flies are hyper, like you in the morning. They sleep all winter long. Then when the spring sun tickles their feet to wake up, they start going crazy."

I always interrupted about this time with an urgency to express to my father, the kind and compassionate side of my character. I would tell my father that I never in my whole life killed a fly. Roaches and mosquitoes - yes, but never did I ever smash-kill a fly.

He always made a point to acknowledge my selective kindness. "Good girl."

"Well, the flies would talk to each other and the word got around. Mornings was the time then all the flies in the room could audition. After about three or four hours of workin', a whistle would tell us it was time to stop what we were doing and open our lunch buckets. That's when all the flies got real serious. It was their last chance to show me how well they can fly. They would do nose dives, back flips, tumbles, twisters and serpentines."

My face showed more seriousness in listening. I knew we were getting close to the good part.

"First, I cleared my work area. Then I took out the paper napkin from my lunch bucket, laid it open on my table and cut long thin strips, about… so wide."

My father would raise his arm out of the water, put his thumb and index finger close together and raise them an inch away from my nose. It took both my eyes meeting in the middle to see the tiny smidgen of space between them.

"After I cut, I donno, about ten, maybe fifteen strips, I would lay them down on my table side-by-side. Then, starting with only one strip, I lay it alone in the center of square sheet of paper on my worktable. On one end of the strip, at the tip I put the tiniest spec of glue "

I was quite satisfied. This was the long version of the story. My father continued:

"Now I had to be extra smart. I start to look around the room, lookin' for the best and biggest fly. And there were plenty to choose from. When I found the fly that appeared to be exceptional, my eyes would follow him closely to make sure he was the best one. Then I would swing my hand quickly in the air and in one quick sweep, catch him in the cup of my hand as not to squeeze him."

My father swung his wet hand in the air re-enacting the capture. Bubbles from the sink followed him and flew off his hand into the air. Splats of suds and water hit the wall, spilled over the counter and dripped down to the floor. I loved the theatrics and the mess that I knew would make my mother mad.

"The winning fly was so shocked and excited he was picked that he would lay in my hand speechless. Then I would gently pick him up with my pocket tweezers and put his belly on the sticky end of the paper strip."

The first time I heard the story I would cry for the flies. Papa assured me that the thin paper napkin strip fell off their bellies after a time. They were never hurt or in pain. He told me it was fun for the flies. Riverview fun and I knew about Riverview. It was the largest amusement park in Chicago and probably in the world. There was 'The Bobs.' the most terrifying rollercoaster that went 87 feet in the air, plus it had 20 rollercoasters, a water carousel, 'Shoot-the-Chutes', and a parachute splash. No one I knew died at Riverview or left there unhappy. I felt better about the flies and pushed away the tears from my eyes.

He continued with his story. "It would take my little fly a couple a minutes to come out of being shocked. I watched him very carefully, waiting for him to give me the sign that he was ready."

I never heard the part about the fly giving my father any sign. I heard this story again and again and never had Papa mentioned 'the sign'. Sometimes he changed things around or added a little more information. My mouth felt glued shut to asking questions.

"Big Mike and some of the other guys moved their stools over to my table to get closer. Leo had already turned on his transistor radio to playing good fly-diving music. The whole department got quiet. Duke Ellington was getting ready to play '*The Mooche*'.

Papa stopped and looked straight into my eyes. "I looked at Leo, Leo looked and me, then we both looked at the fly."

I saw it all in my head even though I never met Leo or the fly.

Papa continued, "I watched the fly. He looked good. I swear Suzka, I never told this to anyone but that little fly winked at me. He was ready."

My eyes were stone-stuck on my father - my head was thinking *Holy Shit!* I learned *Holy Shit* from Stacey.

No matter how many times I heard this story my head thought it new every time.

"I tightly held on to the edges of the paper and tossed the fly to the sky. It was the most beautiful thing. The fly flew up in the air higher and higher then plummeted down and circled back up. His paper tail followed every turn and dip. He flew above our heads, orbiting the room like a shooting star."

For a second I saw stars in my father's eyes. He was so happy.

"Sometimes I would catch five or six flies and have them all flying around at one time. We'd sit there eating our sandwiches and drinking our sodas under a galaxy of shooting stars, dancing comets and Duke Ellington. No one said a word. It was a beautiful thing."

Our eyes turned inward to watching the comet flies in our heads.

My father lifted me out of the sink and set me down on the linoleum. I turned around and leaned my back against his legs for balance and kicked up each leg for the towel wipe-down.

"The end. Now go put on your pajamas. I'll make popcorn for you and your sisters."

I loved footbaths and Flying Comets.

Lil'Vi, my baby sister, loved popcorn more.

Mira, my taller sister was too big and too cool for footbaths and fly stories but she did love popcorn.

19.
D M V

"Over there." A man with a dark face pointed to a ticket dispenser that spit out numbers. He was an oddly suspicious looking character pointing as if he were giving me insider information not available to others. "You gotta take a number. Everybody's gotta take a number."

My mother moved in closer as if she were getting access to non-public information. It all sounded illegal and naughty which piqued my mother's attention.

"Hurry. Listen to the man. Go get a number Suzka. Get two numbers."

"Mom it doesn't make difference if I take two. They're calling the numbers in numerical order."

"Listen to me. Just take two numbers. Why must you always argue with me?" My mother must have fought with her dementia, her old ways won.

"Ok. Ok. I'll take three."

"You're being a sassy smart-aleck, a wisenheimer. Well, go get me four then."

Our number was 424, 425, 426 and 427. I looked up at the 'Now Serving' box, digitally flashing 277.

This was my mother's birthday month and the month her driver's license would expire. She was more confused these days. Sometimes she couldn't remember my name or how many children she had. But she knew the expiration date on her driver license and it had all the signs of being its last and permanent expiration.

It was bitter sweet. This could change everything. But she was exceptionally alert this day as if she studied her sanity all night long. Her wits were to be tested. The stakes were high.

[The contents of my mother's voice regarding
driving and the DMV had three classic themes:
 # 1. "I've been driving since I was twelve."
 # 2. "I'll give the man one, no two bags of candy.
He might need convincing. My eyes aren't that good."
 # 3. "I don't need the photo so maybe
he can just add all that savings onto my score.
I plan on cuttin' the face from my old license
and super glue it right on top of the new one.
It is such a good picture of me."]

My mother loved driving but she drove like a maniac for as long as I can remember. Her specialty was expressways with high traffic volume and mazes of overlapping ramps. But she had that touch, like Picasso with a brush, to switch lanes with swift energy, speed and daring excitement.

"And when they call me to.... well, just move away from me, go over there and read or draw or do whatever you do.... And don't call me 'mother'. If you need to speak, call me by my name, *Violet*." Looking closer she added, "Is that paint on those pants?"

I am not all sure of how to interpret her request. It was hard to be sufficiently objective. I didn't know by what manner I learned to interpret the difference in *Violet's* attitude, which she verbally expressed by the omission of 'mother' when I was to speak of her. But slowly and profoundly I became aware she was different.

"Yes '*Violet*', it is paint on my pants."

I looked around. The room was huge. The floored linoleum was taped with lines, directional lines; a complex puzzle of paths for the numbered to follow. The tape ended at counters where everyone needed to go eventually. No one followed the linoleum's advice. Everyone moved around willy-nilly.

The room echoed every sound, every chair that scraped the floor, every shuffling shoe and dragging walkers as well as all the windowed conversations. Some people trembled and made wheezing sounds. Old people alarmed at being banned from driving forever sat quietly afraid to think of it too loudly.

"What-cha-say? I can't hear you."

A muffled tone-less voice came from an intercom set in the walls. "Now serving 333 at Window A12." The overhead box flashed the neon numbers 4 times and then stuck in place.

"Let me go tell them I'm a senior citizen." My mother, who I refer to as Violet from here on, leaned up from the chair, " I'm gonna go and talk to them. You go get more candy from the car. Don't forget, one bag of the sugarless."

"Sit down… Violet."

"Oh Lord, look at that poor dear."

A man wobbled to the window like a bulldog. He had no neck and wore thick glasses. His frame was round, his toes turned out. He looked like an old dog with worms.

When he got to the window he was nervously excited and could barely see straight.

His wife next to him said "Come on now. Pull yourself together. You can't read it correctly if you're in a frenzy. You got to do some hard brainwork. You got to concentrate on that chart. You got to think with your eyes, all your limbs and any young boy brains you have left over." Her tiny hand clutched the bulldog's hand.

"Lady step back. You are not supposed to help him. He has to do this on his own." The voice came from a thick black woman with large breasts smashed into her DMV's vest. She had noticeably layered lashes heavily glued in place and wore perfume that traveled around as if it was on tour.

"I'm not giving him the answers." The little wife said.

"Just move back."

The man took another extended squint at the chart and uttered a cockeyed screwed up sound. "Ffff-pee. Toz le-ped. Pec-fed."

The DMV agent said "English, sir. Just speak English and read the chart." She spoke sharply with a distaste for foreigners, old or new.

"I'm trying to but I don't speak this DMV crap. Give me an English chart."

"This is the chart you need to read sir. Don't get sassy with me. Just read the letters one by one."

"Ffff-pee. Toz..."

"Letters! They're letters not words! Read each letter separately."

"F-in P...

"Just spell out the word sir. Spell the words for me."

On the other side of the room a uniformed man walked in with a clipboard. He had German features. A striking man astonishingly like what you call 'modern art' in many respects; distorted features, not proportioned but viciously honest. All his parts appeared to be middle-aged. Following him was an older man talking to his wife who met him at the door.

"It was awful." he said. "That guy confused the hell out of me every chance he got; *turn right, turn left, park here, watch out, don't hit that kid.* I didn't see no kid. He made it up to make me crazy. He's not working for our side." His wife listened and didn't say a word. "That guy's a communist. It was awful, Betty. This country's going to hell in a hand basket."

He had failed his test for sure. His nose was as red as a dried beet and his voice sounded like a frantic dog locked in a car. This was an irreparable loss. "Common let's go home. I'm driving." Betty could only follow her angry husband.

Violet and I watched the man and his wife walk into the horizon.

The German inspector separated the crowd as he moved closer into the room. When he felt his presence was noticed he stopped. From his back pocket he took out a sparkling white handkerchief and wiped over his dark mirrored glasses.

I felt cold hands down my back, hands of the inevitable.

"Mrs. Violet! Is there a Mrs. Violet here?" His words loudly cut through all the other noises moving around in the room.

Violet pinched her cheeks and ran her hand over a few loose hairs around her ears before she raised her hand like a little girl in school. "I'm here. You hooo! ...over here. I'm Violet." Waving her entire arm in the air drawing attention to her location. She was ready.

In one sweep she ripped the canvas bag of candies off my arm and innocently moved quickly to her executioner.

"I'm Violet officer."

"I'm not an officer ma'am, I am your examiner, George."

"Yes... but I don't need to be examined." She shook her body and rolled her shoulders. "I feel great. I've been driving since I was twelve."

"Are you ready to drive for me today?"

"Oh yes indeed." They slowly started to walk together out the building to the testing area. "And how are you today, George?"

She paused herself. "You look so much like my son."

[I have no brothers.]

She used her old woman's voice, a gay voice with endings dripping in honey. As she spoke she wrinkled her forehead and animated her cleverness.

"I'm fine Violet, thank you. It's a beautiful clear day. Let's start." George smiled exemplifying his authority.

He turned toward me, "Is she your mother?"

"Yes."

"We'll be back in twenty minutes."

I thought my mother at that moment was moving away from this life. She appeared smaller and seemly more frail than this morning. I thought the proportions in her face were all wrong. Her nose and her ears were bigger. And as she walked away from me I noticed she had a bit of a hump on her back. I never noticed that before.

"Are you diabetic?" Violet asked George.

George bent his body and disappeared into the car.

As they drove away they left me a sky of blue, a sooty blue like an over-painted watercolor. Clouds hung down like cobwebs and drifted slowly as not to be noticed by any gusts. A few knobs of trees and framed houses popped up close together which made everything seem flatter.

I stepped back and leaned against the building. The sun covered my body and made everything sweet and warm as the inside of a dish cover. But I was still worried. It's dangerous to be compassionate when you need to be sensible.

[She Passed !#@%]

Who said that? I looked around and saw George talking to me. What did he say? Did I hear him correctly?

"She passed."

I looked at Violet and noticed a similar surprised look on her face, but she wouldn't let on. She kept her secret well hidden.

George continued talking as he signed and stamped the necessary paperwork

"Well, she drove better when she used her purse to sit on. You'll need to make sure she sits on a couple of cushions when she drives. I'm gonna pass her this time but..."

I heard nothing else after his 'but'.

How did this happen? How could they issue her a license? Well let's just drop licenses out of the sky for everyone. Blank licenses. Let people fill in their names with crayon and draw a happy face in the picture box. Let everyone drive, little babies, blind people, dogs and cats, elephants... I was dumbstruck.

Violet broke my stupor and started talking.

"Common now let's go home. I'm driving. You know, George is really a very nice man. He's Jewish. Married. You want to go to Crystal's for lunch?"

"I don't know mom. I think I... I just don't know anything anymore."

< UNITED AIRLINES >
FLIGHT: #6296 Tues Feb 28
DEPART: Chicago at 1:49 PM
ARRIVE: California at 11:55 AM
CANCELED
Rebook return flight.

STAGE THREE

SYMPTOMS

Changes in behavior. .
Increase in forgetfulness and
confusion with a chain of events.
Wanders. Lost if not supervised.
Help needed to get dressed
and with toileting.

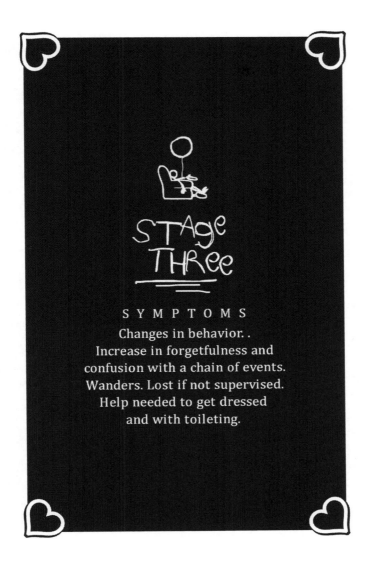

20.
SETTLING IN DEMENTIALAND™

Violet walked about the house gathering things prudently as if she were an archeologist collecting fragile bones from the past. Carefully she bagged what she thought important and moved them into a back room with the tall windows. Daily excavations were unexplainably part of her routine.

In one of her early gathering expeditions, I had noticed she had in her bag a collection of toiletries, a postcard from my older sister with Winslow-Homer-like palm trees on its face, a few rolls of duck tape and a cigar box filled with pennies. Inconspicuously, she then took the collection into the back room and hid them in the freezer, buried a few pieces under cushions and stuffed others in corners previously sworn to secrecy.

I watched her discretely and found myself confused and at times moved by her foresight. It was as if she was moving cross-country, leaving the details of her past behind and relocating to the one room that I respectfully called Dementialand.

I never questioned her doings nor returned any of her collectables to their proper place. I thought her 'brilliant' but had no understanding to why.

[The idea of disassociating from one's surrounding was rather clever on my mother's part without her notice.]

The new surroundings kept my mother detached from the outside world as though she was sitting in a moving train looking out at a passing world with flashbacks to places she once lived and visited from a time she can't remember.

She was growing outside herself, outside the fit of her opinions and beliefs. Her head's collection of facts, dates, faces and fading black and white memories were disappearing. Complete thoughts were cut into pieces. A tiny mosquito armed with the game changer, shot my mother with meningitis-encephalitis. The surface of her life crumbled but in its rapture uncovered the person my mother inherited eighty years ago.

[The following eight hundred words, gives a more forensic description of Dementialand.]

Dementialand was located in the back corner of my mother's house - a room about 15 x 25 feet with tall windows that stood shoulder-to-shoulder and extended from corner-to-corner-to-corner. The windows gave a panoramic view of an outside world - a world that my mother Violet was becoming more and more the least bit interested in, except for the birds that would sit on branches and chat with her about their day. Lace curtains covered parts of the windowed blinds. The curtains and blinds worked together to soften the bold intrusion of an outside world. When the windows were open and the blinds were raised, the outside blew the visiting ghosts of dead relatives into the curtains.

My mother owned the house. Everything belonged to her; the building, the furniture, the 47 Jesuses (one church-like sized) and the garden with plastic planted begonias. She bought it with my father years before death moved him out. Now she was alone. Noises from their bickering had peeled themselves off the walls and left slowly; they had been replaced with the radio weather announcers and game show hosts who argued less with my mother. My sisters and I called her daily, almost, but never at 6:30 on weekdays.

There were very few remaining signs that Pavel, my father once lived there. In a back room, under a glass top of an old dresser, there was a rather impressive but unconnected collection of cards and clippings that he saved for some unknown reason. The collection included three or four photos taken of family members he actually liked, old newspaper articles on unrelated topics, and a number of scattered holy cards back side up showing the stats of a family member that passed away. Everything was pressed, preserved and squeezed under glass like specimens of a scientific study on display: a carefully acquired collection that was telling Pavel's story to no one listening. The gathered group made the glass lay 'drunkerdly' on the top of the bureau.

And there was the photo of his mother Agnes who was living secretly in the top drawer of an old nightstand. No one opened that drawer. Her loving son was her only visitor. After living there for nearly sixty years, the photo aged like any mother would. It grew wrinkled and frayed at the edges. The woman inside the top drawer would eventually disappear forever and no one would ever know. On her back, odd-looking letters were scribbled. Maybe it was a note for my father, her youngest son. I always believed it was. My father showed the photo only once to me when I was young. I walked in the room with the nightstand and saw him weeping. No words were spoken. The air barely took a breath. I remember being too frightened to ask questions or touch the picture. I was little then with big thoughts of finding places to explore and stake a claim for my latest creative dig.

The most visible sign that my father had once lived there was that chain and two-by-four contraption at the front door. It was my father's creation, a foolproof security system. A long heavy chain with metal loops wrapped several times around the knobs of the front double doors. The doors never before seriously locked themselves properly. Anyone with the least insignificant amount of body weight could open them with the slightest shove. For backup, a two-by-four was anchored tightly between the door and a stair railing about six feet away. My father would tell my mother, my sisters and myself and anyone who would listen, *"John Dillinger himself couldn't break into this house."* My mother would always remove the chain and the two-by-four when she knew I was coming from the airport in the middle of the night for a week's visit.

But Violet performed most of her official Dementialand duties from the couch that sat in the middle of the room. The couch that originally belonged to her mother with the tiny pink flowers, green leaves and family secrets embroidered into a faded white fabric. During the day, Violet would sit on the couch and talk with the visiting birds that would be chattering on branches. Jealous leaves tapped on the windows trying to butt in and get her attention. Occasionally Violet would be pushed to look beyond the birds and the leaves to an outside world where a suspicious neighbor was doing questionable things. That will come later.

The house was actually large. Rooms legged out from a long hall like a centipede. Some legs led to more legs leading to smaller rooms. Violet could easily get lost, possibly forever, or possibly she could fall into a rabbit's hole. So she kept herself safe in one room.

[This ends the eight hundred word description of Dementialand]

Everything was more alive in Dementialand. Everything jumped, howled and vibrated. It shook us silly and at times slapped all of us senseless until the last hinge that held all of us tightly to yesterday's yesterday, snapped. I saw my mother's stubborn pigheaded ways cower under the room's furnishings that tried desperately to reupholster time. The days often turned on us and went in and out of their calibrations. All the clocks threw their hands in the air in war-weariness and deserted their posts. The mornings goofed around with the evenings, afternoon often showed up for breakfast and the sun worked for the moon at night. Days and nights had no regard for order. My mother felt she had no choice but to keep herself dressed for all the hours.

Violet was Dementialand's principal resident and crowned head-of-state. All fantasies bowed down to her.

*

My official move into Dementialand was slow and cautious. It took a few months before I could get myself to unpack the clothes out of my duffel bag and put them on hangers. I could not get my head around those very words *'she cannot live alone'*. My head was slammed shut. Every muscle and bone in my body waited for some kind of confirmation. I avoided telling myself almost the truth.

[Gulley Jimson told me
that when you get into one of these spots,
you have no choice but to think like a painter.
He told me that even the worst artist
that ever was, a cross-eyed mental deficient
with the shakes in both hands,
about to paint the first stroke, looks at
the blank canvas as an adventure.
This was a fresh canvas.]

Yes. This was my fresh canvas! And I also told myself that I needed to change my thinking before the first problem shows its devilish face. If not it could be hell for the term of my stay.

I needed to let go of everything from my past; my opinions and old scenarios. Surprisingly enough, it also meant that I needed to let go of everything I thought I was suppose to be.

I settled myself into an open room on the lower level. It was a non-room by conventional standards. No doors, just passageways. Boxed items no longer fashionably acceptable or useful were lowered to this level. The room was close enough to hear the goings-on of my mother and her travels in the night.

21.
DEMENTIALAND'S GADABOUTS

[They lived with us. Maybe
there were twenty or more.
At one time I counted 28.]

It started with one airhead, a huge round blue balloon with a wide black smile. Popping out from the top of its head were two black eyes painted on transparent eye sockets. The balloon was filled with helium and held in space by a thin gift ribbon that was clipped to the magazine rack at the grocery's checkout counter. A card attached to his rubberneck read SKU 44678. I couldn't resist buying it. It looked as if it could pick you up, suck you out of yourself and carry you away; away from computers, canvases and slippery couches with unruly fallen sheets; away from mothers, mosquitoes and the dementias.

I brought SKU number 44678 home and pulled him by his long gift ribbon into the back room. He was hesitant at first and dawdled behind. I had to drag him most of the way. He eventually settled down, looked around at his new home and landed his eyes on my mother.

At first mom was a bit taken aback by the large blue helium gift. She squeezed her face together and stared at the ballooned face then quickly snubbed her head back to the window. She talked with a couple of birds that sat on an outside branch. "My daughter is a crazy person bringing into my house such silliness as if we were having a birthday party for a five year old baby child. It's not my birthday and I am no damn child."

"It's a gift for you mom. I thought it would brighten up the room a bit and make you smile."

"Why do you waste your money to buy such silly things?" My mother ignored the smiling balloon and waved her hand frivolously in the air.

"You can take him back now."

"Mom, it's a gift. I bought it for just for you. His name is... SKU...? Come on now, he's kinda cute, don't you think so? I love his color. You love blue don't you?'

Pause.

“He talked to me when I was in the check-out line at the grocery. He said... *Suzka! Suzka take me home to your mother, Mrs. Violet.*"

I looked directly at my mother. “True. That’s word-for-word what he said.”

"Now you're sounding like your father."

My father always used those same words when he brought home stray dogs. According to my father, homeless dogs, particularly the dogs in pounds, would jump on the cage doors and ask my father to take them home. All the pets we had at one time talked but never spoke a word after my father brought them home and they became part of our family.

"Don't tell me that goofy balloon talked to you. You are a crazy child. And what kind of a name is SKU?"

She looked at me and shifted her eyes closer to the wide smile on the balloon. “You wasted your money. Take him back.”

"You talk to birds and you got the birds talkin' back to you.”

"Birds are God's living creatures. Anyone can hear their speaking. They have little mouths with little voices inside.” She sunk her head into her shoulders and added tiny gestures to her reasoning. “I see them talkin' right in front of my ears. They talk in chirps and tweets and I talk back to'em in whistle and words too sometimes. We understand each other. I don't know why I'm even talking to you about such things."

"Mom, give the poor guy a chance. I think he's one of those Muppet characters. He looks like the Cookie Monster."

I moved SKU 44639, aka the Cookie Monster balloon, at the end of the couch in full view for my mother and any visitor to see. A long string attached to a metal weight in the shape of a heart kept him grounded.

The funny-faced balloon settled in the air and looked directly at Violet. *"You must be Miz Violet. Hello, let me introduce myself, I'm Cookie."*

After receiving no response whatsoever, the room's air drifted the ballooned head toward me, *"She dahn't talk much, dahhz she?"*

Something changed when Cookie was around. He brought a lightness into the room, a soft feather dancing in the cloudy fog. This funny-faced balloon began to make his presence in the room. As we walked around throughout the day his popped-up eyes seemed to have followed us. I started to like the little character. He made me smile. He made everyone smile. My mother kept her distance and talked to the birds about Cookie.

Pretty soon balloon bore more balloons until they formed their own community. After Cookie came Hello Kitty, Dora, Betty Boop and Princess Belle. Then I brought in a couple of Elmos, Tweedy Bird and a few Happy Faces; butterflies, stars and hearts visited on holidays. They were all large in size, their heads measuring as much as three feet in diameter. Ribboned legs determined their height as well as their position.

They moved left to right, turning around and rubbing against each other on invisible drafts. Their flight was engorged by helium. Weights in their shoes kept them somewhat grounded but did not prevent them from scooting closer to Violet, dragging their heart-shaped anchors behind them. Such queer heads lived with us.

The ballooned airheads were the first squatters that moved into Dementialand. They comfortably scattered themselves about everywhere.

Balloons are funny creatures. I learned to love and appreciate their queer ways. They are able to float and skate above everything hard. Only a soft gift ribbon attached to heart-shaped weights, keeps them from running away. But if they wanted to, they could escape and take you with them to a place where everyone is in love and flowers pick themselves.

BALLOON STATISTICS

[A 34" latex balloons filled with helium will generally last between 3 to 5 days. and possibly an extra day when treated with Hi-Float. Foil balloons - 5 to 7 days. In Dementialand, balloons were regularly replaced with their likenesses when needed.]

*

Window blinds once closed, opened their eye slats letting the outside in. Neighbors lined up watching. They turned their faces towards the parade of new residents moving into Violet's house. Some they recognized from standing in lines at the Jewel Grocery; funny looking characters tied to the displays by thin gift ribbons. Women recognized some of the characters from Saints' medallions hanging down at their throats.

Men shook their heads and turned their eyes away in puzzlement.

"I heard Violet's daughter from California moved in with her."

"Isn't she one of those artist types?"

"I saw her once... a funny looking girl."

"Ohhhhh."

"I hope Violet will be ok."

"We can only pray."

"That's all we can do."

22.
RE-ENFORCEMENTS

Those words: *"Your mother cannot live alone...rapid dementia... watch your mother 24 hours...do you understand?"* I wasn't sure what I said at that moment. I vaguely remember hearing something said at the hospital. *"Do you fully understand the seriousness of your situation? Your mother will soon need care 24-7. You cannot do this by yourself... you need to hire a caregiver to help you."*

*

I walked into the back room with the tall windows where the little grasshopper (my mother) sat in her wheelchair.

"Mom, this is Sovina."

The sky had gone to scarlet behind my mother. Slowly she scratched her head not sure who this strange Sovina woman was in front of her and what she might have had up her sleeve. Violet nonchalantly returned her arm to a fold and slyly hand searched for the reassurance that her purse was at her side. Her eyes darted straight ahead at my intentions.

Before she had a chance to speak, I presented my case.

"Mom, you know how crazy busy it has been around here, what with all we both have to do. Well, I have given this much thought. You're an independent woman. I think what you really need is your own secretary, a *kinda'* secretarial day planning helper but also with caregiving skills."

She prepared her face, a wooden fixed smile, which expressed nothing perfectly.

"And what are you gonna do all day, missy? Are you planning on leaving me?

"Oh no, no. I am definitely not leaving."

That was when she abruptly changed the direction of her thought and stared me down. She took what was left in her head and notably asked me, "Who are you?" It was only on an occasion, not very often, when the dementias messed with her head and nagged her to ask questions like '*Who are you?*'

"I'm your daughter, mom." I regretted saying that so quickly, the daughter part.

She looked at me bewildered. She continued staring as if she no longer recognized my face. It was as if she kept hearing over and over again, *my daughter, my daughter, my daughter,* until 'daughter' had no meaning and became just a vibrating sound in her head. It was of little importance really, daughter, mother, sister, brother. They were just words. And in all seriousness, I don't think my mother nor I gave much thought to our connection. I had disembodied that mother-daughterness months ago.

MOM

[Mom – the sound.
A sound involving little more than pressing
your lips together, holding them that way for
a second and then resonating out a puff of air.
A cosmic sound or a mystical syllable
or simply an affirmation to something
divine as in 'om' – acknowledging
our connection to all living beings,
nature and the universe… mom]

That is when the music from the boombox in the other room started. I must have set the timer earlier in the day. Violet came back from her leave. Her head corrected herself and returned her eyes to that of an eagle. “What are you staring at?”

“Nothing. Nothing. I’m not staring.”

“Hello Mrs. Violet. I am Sovina.”

I tried to return comfortably to where I left my thoughts. “I'll be working over there on the dining room table. See my computer and those stacks of papers?" The table had piles of my mother’s past due bills, bank statements, titles and policies and various papers of importance that I had found in overstuffed boxes tucked in her life’s corners.

The room paused while the word *secretary* passed through Violet's head. I played with my ear and bounced my earring around with my thumb, a nervous habit of mine.

"… but we don't need anybody if you’re staying." Her words moved slow and wandered out into the room looking for a place to set while avoiding Sovina’s presence.

Everything told me to wait a second and just hold on. Acceptance was around the corner… it was just a matter of time.

Her face softened as if she were calculating the sound of... a woman with a private secretary.

I thought myself to be quite clever at that moment. Resistance was weakening.

She raised her eyes with a look of surrender. Slowly, Violet spoke with authoritative importance and humble understanding. "Ben MetLife has a sec-terry."

“Matlock, mom... Yes, Ben Matlock also has a secretary

Breath. "Ok now." I placed my hands together and sealed the deal with responding, "Well this feels right. Indeed. Amen indeed."

My mother looked acceptingly serious at Sovina. "You're not into voodoo or anything like that, are you?"

We had other caregivers in the past months. Their memories although not remembered in any detail, if they are remembered at all by my mother, remained in the room, stuck to the walls like old cigar smoke.

<u>Previous Caregiver</u>: Fiona.

Fiona was barely 5 feet tall, 40ish, single, Scandinavian, stout with a double chinned midriff and thin suffering blond hair tied with a red rubber band into a pitiful ponytail. Her eyes matched her hair. She had an ageless face and little whiskers on her chin that made her look like a goat, a young goat.

JOB DESCRIPTION: Support in the daily activities for a kind woman with dementia. Assistance with bathing, grooming, dressing and eating; basic companionship and interactive communication required. Caregiver must look out for the physical safety of the patient. No restrictions on food. No need to give medications.

Flexible hours. Car needed. Willing to stay with patient on occasion throughout the night. *Live-In preferred.*

> REASON FOR DISMISSAL: Energy Hovering. Fiona stood over my mother in the middle of one night and nearly scared her to the death. I heard the screaming from downstairs.

"She's trying to kill me! She's trying to kill me!" I ran up the stairs so quickly I dropped my legs twice. When I walked in I saw Fiona leaning over my mother while circling her full arms above my mother's body like helicopters hovering over a hostage confrontation below. She was wearing a new white bathrobe that I gave my mother for Christmas in 1982. Around her waist she had tied a rope, a heavy rope she must have found in the garage.

Violet was hysterical. "This devil woman wants to kill me. She's a little black scorpion ringed with hellfire! Thank God and all the Saints you're here. She's evil. She would have killed me for sure if you hadn't come in to save me!"

I pushed Fiona aside. "What in the hell are you doing?" She was so damn calm it confused the hell out of me. "It's ok. Everything is fine. Trust me. I was following the energy in the room when I noticed something above your mother was stuck. I was trying to release the blocked entities and invite the flow of positive forces to move again more freely."

Violet scooted to the railed edge of her bed clutching the covers to her chin. "Don't leave me here... When are we going home?"

~~Fiona.~~

Previous Caregiver: Eszter.

Eszter was a full 5 foot 10 inches, 50+, a widowed woman. Her body type was similar to Ernest Borgnine. She had shoe-polish-like raven hair that fell to her chin. She had Picasso eyes.

JOB DESCRIPTION: Support in the daily activities for a kind woman with dementia. Assistance with bathing, grooming, dressing and eating; basic companionship and interactive communication required. Caregiver must look out for the physical safety of the patient. No restrictions on food. No need to give medications. Flexible hours. Car needed. Willing to stay with patient on occasion throughout the night. Live-In preferred. No goats. No energy jugglers.

> REASON FOR DISMISSAL: A Missing Rhinestone Hair Clip. Eszter arrived with two suitcases and went home every third day for two days. Something about this woman made me uneasy. I noticed things like jewelry, lipstick and my rhinestone hairclip missing. And some of the monies from the food jar kept in a kitchen cupboard behind the Cheerios box was missing.

I asked her, "So Eszter, how is it working out for you so far?" Her smile was wide, her teeth too nervous to stand straight in their gums.

"Id'z working out fine. Id'z good for me. Your mother iz so sweet. She iz a pleasure to service."

She talked a little bit about herself, her upbringing, her life in Poland and her children who still lived in Europe. She talked about her dead husband who was now living with the angels. The door was opened and I slid into her conversation with ease that I almost felt guilty in what I was about to do.

"My mother has an angel watching over her, also... her father. He was a gypsy man with a great many powers on both sides..."

I leaned over the table and warmly cupped the top of her hand with mine. I felt the handcuffing gesture of connection between us fit nicely into the story. "...if you know what I mean."

"God, he loved my mother...AND still does to this day. From the time he died he never left her side, guiding her and protecting her from anyone who would have harmful intentions towards her. One time a man stole a twenty-dollar bill out of the side pocket of my mother's purse. And that happened in church. Church! A frigin' church for Christ's sake! Can you believe that? You think he'd know better! Well, that guy got into an accident on the way home and ended up in the hospital. He didn't die or anything. My grandfather was not a revengeful man. He just wanted this thief to know that he should have never messed with his daughter... my mother. I think he lost a leg or got paralyzed or something like that. I know angels, especially dead relative angels. They can certainly be wonderful protectors. Insurance."

I was on a roll. Another story followed with barely a breath between. That night Eszter left and never returned. She called the next day and said her daughter needed her and in being a good mother she would have to quit her job and put her child's needs first. For a week I listened to the radio's traffic reports with more interest.

~~Eszter~~.

Previous Caregiver: Elba.

Elba was 5 feet 7 inches tall, 35 and not married. Don't know why she was single, she was very attractive and appeared very approachable. Her hair was auburn, braided close to her skull and gathered in the nape of her neck. Her eyes were dark green like emeralds, clean and polished as if they were precious stones.

JOB DESCRIPTION: Support in the daily activities for a kind woman with dementia. Assistance with bathing, grooming, dressing and eating; basic companionship and interactive communication required. Caregiver must look out for the physical safety of the patient. No restrictions on food. No need to give medications. Flexible hours. Car needed. Willing to stay with patient on occasion throughout the night. Live-In preferred. No energy jugglers. *Criminal background check required.*

REASON FOR DISMISSAL: Sleep disorder. About 3:30 or 4 in the morning, there were loud noises coming from upstairs. I ran into the room and noticed my mother was fully dressed sitting on the couch as if she were sitting on a bus stop bench. In her hand was the remote that she was feverously trying to operate. The TV was blaring.

"Mom, what's going on? What are you doing?"

"I can't get this God damn remote to work."

Without physically acknowledging that I had entered the room, in a loud whisper she added, "Shhh, she's sleeping." She pointed to Elba without turning her head from the business in hand. Elba was sound asleep in my mother's hospital bed next to the couch. This happened twice.

~~Elba~~.

23. SOVINA

Sovina's hair was thick, black and wild, barely kept in check by an elastic band. Her eyes were like jet-black marbles filled with the reflection of gas jets. At first meeting, she looked familiar, as if I'd seen her before. She was painterly interesting, thick, full and colorful like Caravaggio's painting of Mary Magdalene. And there was a fine-ness about her. She could have easily worked in palaces caring for the children and lady mothers of royalty.

Sovina wore two-pocketed shirts with tiny soft patterns and slacks. "Good morning, Mrs. Violet. Are you ready to start the day?" Every word was toned in sweetness.

Sovina was the first one up in the morning. She would help Violet into her wheelchair, take her to the toilet and make breakfast – soft eggs that folded in on each other with smooth walls and one serving of Ensure. While Violet sipped the butter-pecan drink, Sovina would clean Violet's bed. White sheets would billow in the air like winged parachutes as Sovina sang the songs with the words her mother sang to her in Lithuania. Violet sang along. Occasionally the languages met but more often, Violet missed and resorted to mixing in some creative lyrical gibberish.

"What day is it today?" Violet would ask. "Did they name it yet?"

She looked outside the window. Looking to see if her birds were awake. Maybe they knew what day it was. "Should I go to church?"

"If you would like to go to church, Mrs. Violet, we can go. Suzka would take us both."

"No...well... I'm not sure... Why aren't those damn birds up yet?" Violet was good at juggling more than one topic at a time without her own notice. When she finished with the window, she turned her head back to the eggs. Their yellow eyes peaked at her from under their folds. She wasn't sure what to think or why her eggs were so shy.

"Where are your babies?" A question aimed at Sovina.

"They're back home in Europe, Mrs. Violet."

"Oh... " Pausing in thought, "What in God's name are they doing there?"

"They live there."

"Oh..." Often the dementias ambushed my mother's train of thought. It didn't seem to bother her.

"Are you my daughter?"

Violet went on talking, gibberish mostly, asking parts of questions as if a seam gave way in her head and bits of stuffing fell out. When she emptied all her words, the door closed.

[My mother was a seamstress.
Threads in fine colors dangled down from
her crown. When a memory woke up,
it would slide down one of the threads
laughing and calling for her all the way. Her
head would lean over and catch it just before
it slid into the hole and disappear forever.
She would then stitch that memory into a
quilt that would take her away for awhile
– until another memory woke up and
slid down another
hanging thread.]

Sovina was part of a Lithuanian community of women caregivers. They came from neighboring villages before moving to this country. Their mothers and their mothers' mothers knew of each other; mothers who long ago talked about their husbands, their children and gossiped over picket fences. The wives would bring cookies and breads and sausages to other wives when their husbands died. Sovina received their gifts when her husband died.

Sovina was married at seventeen. She met her husband in the village where she lived - a tall handsome man with thick black wavy hair and strong bones. His work had given them a home. His hands were trained to build the kitchen's cabinets, table and chairs where their children would have dinner and talk about their days in school over potato sausages, fried black bread rubbed with garlic and small cakes baked with poppy-seeds. A bottle of Stumbras vodka sat in the middle.

Their lives together were bound, slow and deliberate. He died ten years ago. A terrible accident, that was all I knew. Sometimes the untold tales of the horrific accident lurked in her words and in the catches of her voice. I never asked. I am sure his face was on a family stone just like my father's parents.

Sovina's home was big and bricked in baked bronze stone. She showed me a picture. It faced the Nemunas River, a river that twisted its way through neighboring villages and eventually spilled into the Baltic Sea. It would break away in Sovina eyes when she thought of happier times.

Behind the house was a garden and behind the garden were hills, populated with stories hidden in its White Elms, the Lindens and its Stelmuze Oaks. The hills were peopled by generations of the unborn, the dead and never seen. They carried the myths and legends that squirmed about the night keeping the villagers banded together. Left behind were the rich smells of honeysuckle, asters, jasmine, blue bells, and hemp.

The soul of Sovina's husband with other husbands walked the hills at night as Sovina set her face to the stars, searching out the arms of God. Her future hung in the darkness. A mortgage bank held the home her husband built as well as her life for hostage. Sovina would have to leave her children in the care of family members and village friends and go to the United States for work. All the Sovina's, the immigrant ladies with heavy accents, sent money and clothing back to their families.

Sovina loved my mother.

My mother loved Sovina.

24.
BARBARA THE BARBER

My mother was more confused these days, a secret she kept to herself. She knew certain ways to hide what was going inside of her. She thought like a grasshopper. Grasshoppers were quick, vigilant and one jump ahead of any combative obstructions or questions. You could never catch a grasshopper off-guard. I knew the workings of this little grasshopper. I kept my mother's secret.

It happens to all people with dementia. All at once they are rather quiet and thoughtful; a bit inattentive to all the surface goings-on in front of them. Even their smiles don't have the same meaning as before. They're not sure whether they're laughing or crying and probably don't care as long as they're doing something to trick and ward off the outside interrogators.

When Barbara walked in the room my mother was somewhat taken aback. She was as blank as driftwood with hardly clue who this strange woman was or why she was standing in front of her, but she had learned on her own that it was surprisingly easier to be quiet and nod her head periodically. My mother seemed to know she could leave when she really wanted to, if she was in desperate straights or simply extra confused. Dancing gypsies in her head for sure would take pity on her and take her away to the music only heard by adventuring explorers. Music that my mother danced to sixty years ago on New Year's Eve when she met the father of the children she now can't remember.

Barbara quietly spread around her 'hellos' as if she was the funeral director at a wake, over-emoting every gesture. She winked in my direction acknowledging my presence and walked over to my mother. The oblivious visitor snubbed the crowd of ballooned airheads. Their stretched smiles leaned forward, closer to the visitor in an attempt to reverse the seriousness in the room. The airheads tried to wiggle old pictures of 'how-things-were' out of the lady's head. Princess Bell, Kitty, Dora and Elmo looked at the visitor out of their fixed eyes that wanted to say something.

Belle swayed side-to-side. *"Oh mama, who is this foreign intruder? ...and look at what she's wearing. Good Lord."* Belle was always pretty free in offering uncooked opinions.

"Calm down, Princess. Let's give Violet's visitor a chance to speak." Kitty was the more sophisticated airhead in the room. She moved around if she was floating in a Prada spring runway show.

Dora reluctantly added, *"Ok, ok girlfriend, we'll give the lady a chance. But she better not screw up the mojo we got going on around here."*

The balloons were filled with excessive chatter.

Barbara was a large woman with tiny eyes framed in silver. Her breasts and belly were zippered into a black dress with tiny white polka dots. Her hair was thin and painted copper brown.

My mother appeared more cautious with her words. She was accustomed to any questions tricky visitors would spring on her, especially the silly questions. Such a waste of time looking for suitable answers to questions that would take her back to the flat places where girdles are required and words stayed in their proper order.

She kept her fingers busy fiddling with small glass crystals on her lap. A thin metal chain kept them in line preventing them from rolling away. The chain's end was attached to a metal coin that led to a bangle of a tiny tortured man. She had no idea what that was about, she just like playing with the tiny glass balls. It kept her fingers happy.

"Mom, this is Barbara. She came to visit you."

Barbara mumbled a few words to me as if my mother wasn't present in the room.

Mom sat in her wheelchair like a grasshopper watching her visitor carefully. She put all the physical features of her visitor in her head hoping to find a match but her thoughts were inpatient. *Barbara, do I know a Barbara? Barbara, Barbra, or did she say barber. BARBER! Oh God in heaven, the woman's a barber?*

[My mother had a way of accessing
the energy of the people around her.
There was no need to know their name,
who they were or how she knew them.
She didn't recognize their surface.
She went much deeper.]

Violet slowed down like a train approaching its last station. Seriousness grew inside her. She was fully aware of the workings of barbers. They could leave you close to baldness if you let them. Barbers had tools, all types of instruments, up their sleeves. They had clippers. Some ran on automatic and if not in the hands of an experienced barber, they could mow over a head relentlessly, cutting down every hair in its path.

Violet stared at the barber-Barbara. Her eyes were on their knees pleading; *I beg of you, don't chop off my hair. I like my hair.* Violet squinted her brain tightly in place.

She cannot wander. She must stay here and keep both her eyes fixed on the barber-Barbara.

Violet, deep in thought and deep in her stare, worried about other possibilities. Maybe this barber-Barbara will cut into her head... taking stuff out and replacing them with events that never happened. *How barbaric. What kind of a woman is this? Has this woman no shame!*

The visiting woman, a Barbara with an undisclosed profession, squatted down spreading her cherub legs apart. She carefully wobbled her balance using the handles of my mother's wheelchair. The barber-eyes squinted. One eyebrow moved up leaving its twin a bit confused. Barbara's face was questioning her own expression. *Are we sad, are we happy, what's going on here?* A face just needs to know what to do.

She looked all about my mother like a detective at a crime scene. Putting a stare on this little grasshopper comparing her to pictured images she had in her mind's hand. Old pictures taken from a time when they first met years ago before Violet ever got confused. She looked for the tight French twist, pearled necklace and Italian shoes. Barber-Barbara held on to the past very tightly. She lived in old albums and carried them with her wherever she went. Barbara could not see what was in front of her - she could only see what wasn't there.

Violet stood tall sitting in her wheelchair. Her ballooned friends were near, protecting her the best they could under these circumstances.

Princess Belle scooted closer to Violet for support. "*Stay calm Miss Violet. We got your back, baby doll. We ain't going nowhere. This lady barber don't intimate me none. She'll have to deal with me first before she even thinks about touchin' a hair on your pretty lil' head."*

AN UNSPOKEN TRUTH

[Violet never talked directly to the airheads as she did with the birds. But I believe on occasion she acknowledged their presence with bridled fondness.]

Barbara started asking questions with facial contortions. She raised her voice and extended her neck for clarity. Before Violet could put the jumbled words into sentences, before she could figure out what this woman's face was saying, the woman would ask another question. Maybe it was the same question, Violet thought. Maybe she rearranged the order of words as a test, a trick of some kind.

"How - are - you - feeling - Violet ? Do - you - know - who - I - am ? Ann - says – hello. She - is - praying - for - you."

In a lower softer voice, Barber turned her head to me and added, "Well, we're all praying for your mom... and for you of course."

My mother kept squinting her brain. She cautiously lifted her arm so as not to cause any attention. Nonchalantly she stretched her hand to the back of her head making sure everything was just as she remembered. Her fingers shook robustly and then settled on the fine curls at the nape of her neck. *Thank you,*

Jesus, she whispered to herself. Stars flashed in her eyes. She blinked. All worries were lost in her face. She locked her eyes back into themselves satisfied.

Barbara confused herself in finding the appropriate words. She tried to use previous conversations, changing the dates and weather conditions where appropriate and filling in the dry spots with useless current events. Barbara smiled quickly like one who says, *the quirkiness of dementia* but really means *it's a pity.*

Then she lowered her voice, a sign of seriousness, "I hope your mother gets better and returns to her old self."

['HOPE" was exiled from Dementialand.
I hated the word. How arrogant of a word
to make me choose between uncertainty
with its false dichotomies or
to be 'here' in the present moment.
The virtue of hope seemed meaningless.
'NOW' was the all holy.]

*

After the Barbara's visit I moved a number of our ballooned friends to the front door. Visitors entering Dementialand needed to change their pitiful ways, which required in most cases, a major attitude and body adjustment. I staggered a line of balloons from the front door to my mother's room – the kingdom of Dementialand. Their weighted shoes held them in place and staggered them to slightly higher than any visiting callers. When the door opened the breeze hit the line of inflated characters making them sway and bob up-n-down to get the visitor's attention. Not that a bunch of smiling, squeaky large, pop-eyed balloons needed any extra help from the breeze. The collection of latex smiling faces followed each other creating a colorful line of emissaries.

Elmo, the largest balloon in the collection was the first one to address the visitors. *"Hello there, how ya doin'? Welcahm to Miss Violet's home. Just need ta check you in and go over a few things. This ain't no 7-Eleven. Smile please. Want to see those pearly choppers. You gotta' smile. No gettin' around this. And, don't give me no attitude, I wanna see 'happy' spread all over you like sweet butter."*

As the front door opened, everyone was taken aback by the mob of inflated characters. Their wide latex smiles and bulging black eyes strictly enforced a code of compliance to all visitors. No one could avoid the drill.

"I'm going to go over the rules just once, so listen up. First: No pop quizzes, no questions regarding history, biology, physics, or mathematics. Second: No pictures, no albums, all of us here live in the moment. Not much concerned about yesterday's garbage or tomorrow's pick up. Capiche? Third: Violet is not a psychic or a psychologist. Avoid all who-am-I questions. We suggest you reserve those questions for your therapist."

"We don't allow any use of interrogating methods, no yelling, cutting, no water-boarding. If you break any of the rules, we'll rip out your imagination and you'll live out the rest of your life in excruciating blandness with no smelling capabilities. Got any questions? No. Ok, move on."

My mother's callers were speechless. They walked up the steps, facing the ballooned guards one at a time.

"Hey, hey you. What's this? No baggage allowed. Leave all your baggage at the door."

"And you ma'am, in case you don't remember, it's Monday, the president is Obama. Go now and be nice."

The callers walked slowly past the parade of characters pausing by each one as if they were in a reception line at the royal palace. Their eyes absorbed the color and the flight to smaller, younger times. More than often they cracked a cautious grin questioning whether to simply nosedive into the delight of it all.

Two Happy Face balloons were the last in the long line of floaters before anyone walked into the room where Violet was waiting. *"Live in the moment, baby, live in the moment."*

As they entered the room, Violet was sitting in her wheelchair surrounded by her ballooned court. The string holding on to a Smiley balloon was wrapped around the arm of Violet's chair. On one side was Dora and on the other side was Princess Belle. Betty Boop had her back. Cookie was the tallest of all the balloons. He supervised almost everything that was going on in the room. The balloons said barely a word that could be heard. Occasionally we heard a grunt, a squeak but for the most part they tried very hard to keep their opinions to themselves.

We were all pulled into this surreal space, which is what made my mother and this room called Dementialand so alluring – a place where the jasmines were sweeter than ever remembered. And only there, in that room, reality was reordered, reworked and made to show its significant side.

"Do I know you?"

25.
A PHILIP MARLOWE INTERROGATION

Philip Marlowe entered the interrogation room at 11:00 on a morning in mid-October. It was quiet. The air was stale and lay in the corners, slouched against the concrete wall like a wet street dog void of richly breeding. One huge window, stripped down of any outside light, dominated the room. Left of the window was a steel bulky intercom box. Marlowe moved his mouth closer to the mesh screened plate and pressed down on the intercom's button. He spoke into the aperture, which made his words bigger in the adjoining room. "Bring in the suspects."

Marlowe was a man in his late forties, from the late forties, a wisecracking detective. He wore black pants, a white shirt and a thin tired tie. He had dark hair, paper clip eyes and a chin that was too long for his face. He liked liquor, women and working alone.

As he looked through the two-way window, uniforms escorted five suspects into the florescent'ed bright adjoining room. Violet stood close to Marlowe, close enough to smell his Old Spice and the pastrami he had for lunch. Violet felt the dark around her back.

The suspects walked in single file onto a narrow platform. When all suspects filled the platform, they made a forty-five and faced their reflection. Around their necks, thin chains held white cards with black numbers, one through five. The cards covered their breasts. The five suspects also carried small pieces of paper at their side.

Marlowe pulled a metal chair out and offered Violet a seat. The room was black, like the inside of the Cicero Olympic Theater on Cermak Avenue during a showing of the *'The Big Sleep'* with Humphrey Bogart and Lauren Becall.

Violet had a sitting height of 4 feet 2 inches on tippy-toes. Her hair was snow white under a wide brimmed black hat with a bird-caged veil that partially covered her face. She wore a short-pocketed jacket, pencil skirt and a soft crape blouse with tiny pearl buttons leading up to a choir of ruffles around the opened neck. She believed Jewish people make the best doctors and the best lawyers - a thought that came to the front of her head suggesting she might need one.

Marlowe was patient in asking, "Violet, I want you to look at each one of these women and tell me if any of them look familiar. Can you identify any of these suspects as your daughter? Take your time."

Violet slowly moved her attention from one of the line-up ladies to another. "Well, they all look so cute but I'm not sure about the one on the end. She's quite dark. Was my husband black? Do you know?"

"I ask the questions here. Look at the girls carefully. I need your full cooperation right now. Do any of these girls look familiar? Could any one of these suspects be your daughter?"

Violet stayed calm. Her hands were comfortable, folding on to each other and holding on tightly to her purse. They were not going anywhere. Under the weight of her broken, wounded memory was a bright, strong woman and she knew it. "Well... hmmm, I do like Number One."

Marlowe moved back to the intercom box and spoke into the voice box. "Number One step forward and read what's on the paper in your hand." Suspect number one, a slim redhead spoke with volume-forced enunciation as if she were auditioning for a part on Broadway. "Hi mom. I'm *starrrrving*. WHAT...do you have to eat?"

Violet began to feel more confident. Her memory loss was out of her hands and now a police matter. Her head accepted being an integral part of the investigation, working side-by-side with Marlowe. "That one, maybe. She's so pretty. I like what she's wearing. Such a cute dress."

Marlowe's seriousness tore into Violet's eyes. "Are you sure?"

Violet's eyes grew weaker behind her glasses. They were working far beyond her continued attempts to sort through the faded pictures of her past.

Marlowe stared at the little woman, looking for some affirming reaction. He had been in the interrogation business for a long time. He knows what to look for. "Violet, I need you to concentrate. Look carefully."

"Well... number three looks familiar. Maybe it's the shoes. I think I have a pair just like those."

"Number Three step forward and read what's on the card."

Suspect number three, a skinny woman wearing turquoise Sergio Rossi heels, a simple cropped top and a god-awful sequined short skirt that slapped the lights' reflection when she moved forward, read... "Hi, mom. I'm hungry... I mean starving." She dropped the paper to her thigh and looked out into the defeated reflection of herself in the two-way mirrored window. She awning'd her hand out from her forehead... "Can I start all over again? I know I can do better." Her outfit or her Sergio Rossi gave her little confidence.

Marlowe rests one hand on Violet's chair and the other on the table. He continued the interrogation.

"It's..." Violet squeezed her eyes for a closer look at all the suspects, waiting for a spark, a flash, a match. Violet was trying so hard to make out if she knew anything. She would have to rely on her charm and inspiration of the moment. "Number Three... I strongly believe I think it's number one."

"Yes. No. Or not sure?" Marlowe presses again, pinched with agitation.

"Well, if I have to take a daughter, I'll take the Number Three. She looks like she'd be a very nice one." Violet pauses as if she was thinking. "She must be my daughter; she's wearing my shoes. Ok, I'll take Number Three. Are we done? Can I go home now?"

Violet's head floated above her. It was there, all alone. Waiting for a bus, a train, a balloon to take her away to the next thought, to take her away from Marlowe. Violet's head whispered to her... *We're done here!* She got up from her chair, rearranging the grip on her purse.

"Not so fast, missy." Marlowe was not about to let Violet walk away.

"I don't like your manners, Mr. Marlowe."

"And I'm not crazy about yours. I don't mind if you don't like my manners. I don't like them myself. I grieve over them on long winter nights."

Violet sat back down in her chair and changed the direction of the conversation. She traveled to a place where she was comfortable, in control and safe. She silently stared into the windowed suspects and confidently looked back at Marlowe.

"I'd like to buy a vowel?"

DEMENTIA'S HIDDEN GIFT

[This woman had no idea who I was.
She has no idea I was once a smoker,
was thrown out of school twice and a certified
rebel with strong opinions, not remotely shared.
To her, I was new, flawless - immaculate to the bone.
This was all strangely wonderful.]

*

I called the house phone with my cell from another room. Sovina answered and I asked to speak with my mother. My mother talked with her rebellious middle child, living in a converted warehouse 2000 miles away. The living room wall was all that separated our conversation.

"Hi Mom. It's Suzka. How are you doing?"

"SUZKA! Why haven't you called or come to see me? You know your sisters call me everyday and ask how I'm doing. Every day. Did you know Lil'Vi has a baby?"

"Oh, that's nice." My sister's son, my nephew was twelve.

"Did you see him? He lives real close to you, someplace there in California. You must go see him. She sent me pictures."

"Well mom, actually it's a bit of a drive. She lives over 400 miles from where I live."

"That's nothing. I started driving when I was twelve and I drove everywhere. You gotta go and see her. And go see Mira too. She lives out there somewhere. She called me this morning."

After a short breath she continued. "She teaches all day long. I don't know how she does it... You know, both your sisters came to see me last week. Did I talk to you since then? We had a wonderful time."

[Never happened]

"And where were you?" She asked.

"Uh..."

"Did I tell you that two women are living with me now? Did you know that? I don't know how they got here. One is from Europe. She can talk a little Slovak. The other can't talk any European words to save her life the poor thing. She's nice... the other one. She paints on her cloths. She's a strange girl."

The voice changed with serious undertones. A mumbling sound crawled through the phone's receiver. Her words were lowered and felt as if they were cupped into the mouthpiece fearing its intention might be overheard.

"They don't feed me. They don't feed me nothing. I am all skin and bones. Thank God I have my Ensure or I'd be a dead person talking to you right now."

*

Rain was slapping against the window. It was hot and stuffy in the room, too hot for October. I unbuttoned the silk covered buttons from my mother's pink bed jacket. Lightness moved through her like white birds. I thought I could never paint such a face – a face like fine china porcelain; skin like alabaster. The thin coverings over her eyes were tinged with blue. Around her neck hung golden chains strung with crucifixes, medallions of the Sacred Heart and silver metals of the Virgin and other folks. All were Pope-proofed in blessings. Her boned fingers tightly gripped a red gift ribbon that went to the sky lifting her above the dementias. A ballooned happy face at the top smiled at the accomplishment. All the suns and stars kept her grounded in her mystery. Her feet kept quiet and proper.

My mother was asleep somewhere under her skin. This night, the outside failed to sabotage her dreams and destroy her sleep. I watched without a sound in my head. She was close to everything true and simple. There were no pictures sitting on her lap.

[Forgetting involved a series of
self-cancelation and profound awareness.]

*

< UNITED AIRLINES >
FLIGHT: #499 Wed Apr 5
DEPART: Chicago at 10:42 AM
ARRIVE: California at 3:47 AM
CANCELED
Rebook return flight.

Suzka

S Y M P T O M S

Increase in social withdrawal.
Inability to recall names of close family members and caregivers but able to recognize familiar faces.
Confusion and agitation worsen in the late afternoon and evening as the sun goes down.

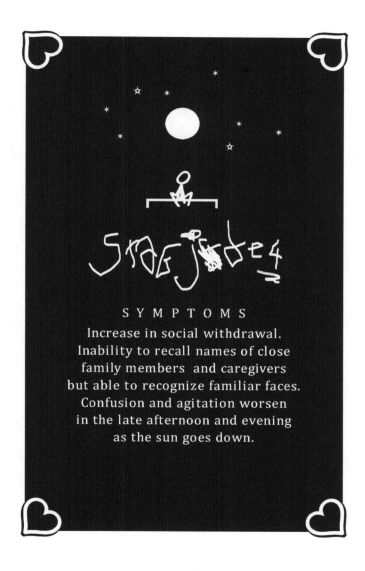

[My mother could un-see
what she had already seen and
un-hear what she had already heard.
I could do that sometimes,
but I had to work at it.]

26.
DELUSIONS
Illusions, Delusions, Hallucinations and Paranoia

Illusions are essentially seeing (most common), hearing, tasting, feeling, or smelling something that is there but perceiving or interpreting it incorrectly. Optical illusions are a perfect example. Illusions are what entertain us at magic shows.

Hallucinations can be understood as a sensory

experience that is imagined. In other words, it's something a person sees, smells, hears, tastes, or feels (or any combination of those). When someone with Dementia has a hallucination it often involves visions of the past and the sense of reliving old experiences.

Delusions are not the same thing as hallucinations. The primary distinction is that, unlike a hallucination, a delusion involves a set of false beliefs despite contradictory information. A person with dementia suffering a delusion may be overwhelmingly suspicious of the people around them, believing that family members or caretakers are trying to trick them and steal their possessions, or that the government or police are following them, or any number of highly paranoid scenarios.

Paranoia is an unrealistic, blaming belief. A person with paranoia will not accept explanations of the unreality of their beliefs. Paranoia can result from damage to the part of the brain that makes judgments & separates fact from fiction. This paranoia is common in people with dementia. Confused people with dementia often misinterpret their circumstances due to a diminished state of awareness and a reduced ability to understand what is happening to them.

["Of course it is happening
inside your head, Harry, but why on earth
should that mean it is not real?"
—Harry Potter and the Deathly Hallows]

27.
THE GYPSY SUNDOWNERS

In the later parts of the night, after dinner, after the day's articles were washed and put away and everyone was asleep. The air quietly began to push aside all the remaining thoughts of order.

The blinds were pulled up and the windows opened wide. A breeze would blow the curtains in closer, maybe to get a better look. The room fell downward from its surface clearing the way for the strange band of sundowners. And it was in those nights, when I often heard my mother mumble gibberish into her pillow so loudly that she would often scare herself. It sounded like all her thoughts were arguing inside her, trying to kick their way out for they were finished remembering and wanted to leave.

The night's replacement carried with them bags of game changing spells; 'gypsy sundowners' I called them. They were memory robbers in the day but at night they were the moon's storytellers bringing tales from the past, fanciful recollections and confessions too. Stories not constrained or limited to any points of views. The gypsies knew that the greatest stories and truths ever told, needed the freedom to breathe on their own.

sundowning *verb. sun'doun-ing*
– disorientation, confusion and agitation;
– changes in the brain of someone with dementia affecting their inner 'body clock';
– trouble separating dreams from reality

*

The air inhaled its staleness and the smell of jasmine filled in the empty space. A sound of trombones traveled through the night. The magical sounds heard only in grand parades, sounds of blessings sprinkling themselves with holy waters. Belly laughs escaped their constraints and flew effortlessly like feathers in the wind. The sundowners paraded in with bells on its feet. Bells not heard by sleeping daughters.

The marching sounds woke Violet. She sat up from her bed and looked around the room. She thought she saw in that moment a light flickering through the dim atmosphere. Not quite sure, she grabbed on to the side-rails of her hospital bed and held on tightly with all her senses. A bouquet of color, rich colors of crimsons, scarlets, lemons and yellows and emeralds burst into the room. Uproariously and without direction, the colors took form.

Violet looked down at Suzka who was asleep on the couch. Maybe this was something she shouldn't share, Violet thought. Maybe this was one of those secrets she would keep to herself. So much was going on in front of her that she didn't recognize nor understand.

Colors spread apart and bloomed into women adorned in rich fabrics of silks and glazed cottons. The women cackled and laughed with each other. With intriguing quandary Violet leaned closer into her vision.

The women were not linked to faces Violet could remember. But she kept her eyes on the visitors and they had their eyes on her too - that's what made them so believable. The women were most vivid and compelling. They looked like they were some kind of performers, maybe dancers. *Why are they here? Are they here for a party, perhaps a wedding that I forgot to remember?* – she might have thought.

Violet was very quiet with her thoughts and careful in trusting the outlandish possibility that the ladies might have come to take her back to her own wedding. Time had its' own mind. She knew to remain quiet and wait in uncertain endings.

Violet locked her body in place. Her eyes did all the moving around the room.

The troupe was not large, about eight women - gypsy women with thick hair, brown and red with purple highlights - hair that curled down their backs to their waist. Their skin was olive in color their lips were ruby red. They had enormous green eyes surrounded by thick lashes. The shape was almond making them look most beautiful and exotic.

They wore large hooped earrings and charm bracelets with hanging silver and gold amulets, polished stone jewels and coins. Their skirts were long, full and flared out whenever they twirled around - borderless skirts with runaway colors. Some wore boots that came up to their knees. Others walked and danced on only bare leathered feet. Their blouses were strawberry red and ruffled along the top stretching from shoulder to shoulder. Their ruffles lowered themselves seductively showing ample cleavages. The visiting women carried brocade and moleskin bags filled with the sounds that gold and crimson would make if they could.

The gypsy women were proud, independent and self-willed women, multi-layered and complex which was their fascination. They were free whimsical women ahead of their time, eternal outsiders to conformity.

It was a bright night. The moon demanded all the attention of the sky and its stars as a conductor would, standing before his orchestra. The night abided and broke apart into specs of crystal flooring where the gypsy women would start their dance.

At first they moved slowly, swinging their hips to the music, moving their arms so freely that their bodies looked like one long wave of maiden-like movement. The copper clapping of their arm jewelry filled the space around them. They created a current of liquid colors - the air followed them and danced in circles. Inside the window's reflection, more dancers were brought into the room.

Violet's eyes moved into their dance. The music bathed in the marrow of her bones. She beamed and felt the power inside her. Everything was loud. She would link herself to the subtle rhythm flowing throughout the universe.

Violet in time loved the gypsies and opened her self to their dance and storytelling.

This night, the gypsies' dance told of a wedding story that took place in Chicago on a hot summer night when the air outside was thick and old; when the sun left slowly, wet and exhausted from the humidity; and when lazy fireflies lowered the sky and talked a bit with the stars. They spoke of a time when large windows in a prominent city pavilion were as open as they could be, begging the outside air to come inside and dance with the music; trees close by just watched – the trees had no rhythm not like the gypsy ladies.

The women held out their hands and helped Violet scoot to the end of her bed where a small opening offered just enough space to escape.

The freedom enticed Violet.

The dancers befriended her and Violet trusted her gypsy friends. She could not remember what they stole, so they were not thieves.

Violet's face changed as she turned all her attention on the dancers with a quiet sharp look.

"I will indeed dance with you." The initial request she felt in her heart.

Once Violet left her bed, once she let go, she moved around the room as if she were floating on her feet. The air romanced itself on oceans of salt, which lightened her load. A natural wonder inside her swayed her hips back and forth and turned her in place.

The gypsies danced around her. Everything was impetuous and unrehearsed. They danced hard, deliberate with spectacular turns and balances - hot blooded and seductive, beautiful and appealing without being vulgar. Their dance was effortless, jiggling tambourines as extensions to their bodies, never loud or aggressive. They danced all their colors outside the lines.

They danced and laughed and continued twirling and spinning around Violet. The gypsy women kept the music going.

I was sleeping on the couch the entire time and never heard the gypsy women but was wakened by a sound, the jingle of bangles. Of course, I was dreaming.

"Mom. Mom, what are you... what are you doing? How did you get out of bed?"

Startled and oblivious at the same time, Violet spun around slowly, paying no serious attention to anything outside the music. There was color and excitement in the room that I never felt before or since. My mother was waving one hand in the air and making tiny steps from side to side. She cupped her arthritic hand, scrunching the bottom of her nightgown in its palm and held it out to the side rolling and weaving it into the air. Elmo danced with Dora, Betty Boop with Cookie and Kitty, the other ballooned airheads swayed back and forth to the music only heard by angels or by the night's breeze from the opened window.

She looked me in the eyes as if she were trying to make out if I knew anything. Her eyes were bright and full, like a new bride, well lined with rich memories stripped of their calendared dates. And at the same time, she was fading away from me. I had to look twice before I could see the only woman I knew as my mother.

Violet was dancing with someone inside of her. Dancing with the muses and the natural rhythm God gave her. Her feet double-stepped hard on the names, dates and information lost in her head. She twirled herself around dancing like a baby swan, young and purposeful.

I could only watch.

[My mother loved to dance. She was the first one on the dance floor with my father at every family wedding. She would have danced at wakes too if they had better music.]

Dementia pursued my mother in the nights. Maybe it was when she danced with the gypsies that it had made up its mind that it was going to have Violet for its own. It wouldn't be easy. My mother had guarded her wits and hid them from the nighttime robbers. But dementia carefully thought this through. It knew it had to be patient if it wanted to have its prize in the end.

Dementia hid behind trees on the side of the night's moons and in dark's empty spaces, waiting for its chance. It would come from behind her quietly and whisper her name. Wherever Violet went she would hear its echo.

Violet disappeared more often, sometimes for only a few seconds, other times for an entire day. In some ways, it was as if she was having an affair. She couldn't hide the change inside of her. The unfaithfulness to status quo, to the norm, to the structure and temples she had built. I noticed her struggling with an unexplainable excitement jumping inside of her and the guilt she must have had that pushed away its promised happiness. It was that scary freedom only a new love brings. The wide freedom so big and so loud it disturbs and whacks everything in its path.

Was my mother holding on to a secret, afraid she might get caught, worried that her new lover would call for her impulsively at any time? How could anyone resist a new love's passion?

I found myself obsessed in wandering curiosity.

Where does she go when she leaves me?

28.
THE AFFAIR WITH SKEETER

Violet stood in a roped line at the border with the long crowd of other travelers. Her black purse was tightly tucked under her arm. Another hand, her own, gripped the purse's side opening for extra protection. She was in full view of the armed soldiers who guarded the border between the official recorded reality and the undocumented realities that took refuge in Violet's head. Faceless inspectors behind tall counters checked all purses for contrabands.

Violet wore a silk-like belted dress in soft white with lavender flowers. Its silky material calmed her girdled body. The girdle's job was to keep Violet and her memories strapped in place - memories she needed; they were her credentials, her identity. Violet took everything she could remember and hid them in the zipped secret pockets inside her purse. She was a careful smuggler. The border inspectors already confiscated her box of Christmas Eve memories; the creamed mushrooms and the milked bread cubes sweetened with poppy-seeds and sugar. They seized the honey that dripped from her father's finger that had marked her forehead with a small cross, a Slovakian tradition smuggled from Europe. The remaining honeys that were later poured on white wafers embossed with pictured scenes of the baby Jesus in the manger were gone.

It was all gone. They took it all.

The inspectors impounded her wedding dress, all her floured recipes, and erased the faces off her family photos. The tall dashing man who once twirled her high above the ground as well as their three birthed babies, gone, all seized. Birthdays, Sundays, presidents and numbers were scrambled and dumped from her memory. Violet watched the inspectors handcuff Jesus and take him to another room. Before Jesus vanished, he turned back and winked at Violet. *You'll be ok.*

"Move to one side. Let us through. Everyone move to one side."

A harnessed dog dragging a uniformed agent behind him sniffed Violet's shoes. The dog sniffed everyone's shoes. Violet pressed her purse closer to her body and watched the nervous dog intensely sniff and drag the official through the line whipping everyone who got in his way with his muscular tail.

A tiny man with baby chin hair and an oversized uniformed shouted out "Next!" His voice was stuck in changing.

Violet scooted to his counter. She forgot to bring a bag of candy, a sweet bribe from a little defenseless lady with age.

"Do you have any memories you want to declare?"

"No."

"Have any pictures, flashbacks, stories." The young inspector slid his elbow further into the counter and leaned sarcastically to ask, "any relative holy cards up your sleeve?"

"Of course not."

The inspector looked over the counter and visually scanned Violet's body, stopping at the black leather purse tucked under her arm. "What's in the purse?"

Violet knew how to play the game. "What, this purse? Are you talking about this silly thing? Oh there's nothing inside. Why, it's not even a purse really. I haven't the slightest idea why I even carry this silly thing around."

The inspector looked into Violet's blank eyes looking for something to give away any secret memories she wanted to keep. He thought of his mother, how she worked as a cleaning lady in an office building at nights for him to continue his schooling. Now he works for the government, a border agent. His mother was proud of her son.

"You look familiar. I might know your mother." Violet's last hope.

"Move on." He let Violet pass but put her on the list of *suspicious characters.*

Violet fooled him. There were thousands of secrets hidden in her purse, secrets and memories that took her elsewhere. She held onto them tightly and kept them to herself. Even God did not know of them.

Violet flattened her hand against her chest pressing down on the giggle jumping inside.

Violet moved quickly past the memory inspectors and followed the crowd into another room; a room large as a school gymnasium and beige, a scuffed beige surface. It was littered with people moving in unruly opposite directions to themselves. The air had no choice but to hold its breath. It was unwilling to move the heavy odors in fear that the room would gag and cough on the travelers. It all smelled like spoiled meat that sat on the counter too long.

Violet walked through the cluttered area of travel toward the metal detector. It would be the final check before she could cross the border. She followed the crowd and funneled herself into the slow line. Sounds behind her reported canceled travel announcements. She never looked back at the lonely place with its suffocating sky. Violet kept her eyes on the line ahead.

A glass wall divided the borders. On the other side Violet saw crowds of people watching the arriving visitors. The glass wall was filled with happy heads on spring necks that bobbled up, down and sideways. Jumping children popped up between the voiceless heads.

In the center of the waiting crowd was an attractive steady-headed man dressed in tall black. Violet couldn't help but notice his striking appearance in the crowd's color. He was statuesque, handsome and mysterious. Violet noticed the man float across the glass. He moved as if he had no feet, gliding toward the glass wall's edge. He mouthed a silent sound of her name.

Violet dug her heals into the ground as the man moved closer to the border's port of entry. Everything in her head argued with her. *What is he looking at? Turn your head away. We don't know this man...* Violet told herself. *Look away and whatever you do, don't let him catch you looking. Turn away. Turn away quickly.* Violet repositioned her purse and fiddled with its straps, a reasonable distraction that kept her mind busy.

Time teased Violet and blindfolded any conventional thoughts. Her instincts moved her torso as far as it could outside the line and straightened her head for a level view. She swept the wall looking for the attractive stranger behind the glass. Suddenly, her eyes hooked into his eyes like a truck about to run into a tree. She snapped back and reprimanded her actions. *I told you eyes not to go there. See what you started. Now he saw you looking. Stop it. Look away. Don't let him catch you.*

The curious admirer behind the glass window softened his face and smiled at Violet's girlish innocence.

The line moved slowly. Violet clutched her purse close to her breasts as she waited for another TSA officer to wave her through the two large metal detectors. She told her eyes to stay close and not to wander off, as small children would often do when traveling with their parents. But her eyes would stray to the side without paying attention. They went to the mysterious man on the other side of the window.

Violet held him in her eyes just long enough for him to notice then quickly looked away disowning her curiosity. Her legs dangled like a marionette whose strings got tangled in play from above by its puppeteer.

He made her nervous. Nervous enough that her first thought was of peeing.

She talked inside her head. *What's he up to? There is something odd about that man. There are layers of purpose in him. I don't know what it is but...* Violet turned direction in the middle of her thought and scanned the walls around her. *I think I need to find a toilet.*

A tall TSA officer waved Violet through. The image of her stranger stuck in her eyes like fresh wallpaper. She walked slowly through the metal detectors as directed. When she reached the middle, fate grabbed her legs. The heel of her shoe got caught on a shagged bathroom-like rug. Her body leaped in front of her leaving part of her behind. The hard floor on the other side was where she was destined to crash, breaking all her bones into sharp chips. As if she were watching an instant replay, the accident's slow motion deepened the terror inside her.

Arms came from nowhere. The wings of an angel in flight caught the falling queen. Her heart raced. White doves flew from the rafters. Sanctified bishops swept their purple garments blessing the air. Violet squinted her eyes in the angel's sunlight. She was mesmerized by words as they floated down on parachutes.

"Are you ok?"

An angel with dark hair caught Violet. His soft curls were loosely pulled back and tied together at the base of his neck. He wore Jesus sandals made by Nike.

His eyes were young and filled with the remnants of laughter. *"Let me help you up."* Her handsome savior raised her gently to her feet. With one arm he held her waist to steady her balance. *"Madame, should I call for help? It looks like you might have injured your ankle."*

Her angel looked into the crowd. *"Is there someone here to meet you...any family, children?"*

Violet pealed her eyes off his face and looked at the area around her. Words left her slowly not sure where to go. "I... I don't know."

The strange angel looked around and noticed that everyone had moved into groups and slowly faded into the walls.

"Then let me be of service to you. My full name is Anopheles deMentia but everyone calls me Skeeter."

The moon, the stars, all the gods in heaven applauded. Fate cleared a way for Skeeter and Violet to walk to a small table with two chairs sitting next to a closed Starbucks.

"I must tell you, until I actually saw you, I had no idea who I was to meet or why I was sent here. Life is so simple. It has a plan for us all."

The language spoken on the stranger's side of the border was foreign to Violet. If only she had her bag of candy to give to the rescuing angel, a small gift of gratitude. Nothing was familiar. Violet called her eyes back and lightly scolded them for talking to strangers.

"Let me get you something to drink. Some water or jasmine tea perhaps." Without waiting for a response, he helped Violet into a chair. *"Which do you prefer?"*

“Oh no, nothing for me. I have Ensure in my purse. Maybe I'll take a tiny sip of that to steady my nerves."

They spent hours together talking, nearly an entire afternoon. Violet leaned closer into herself and talked of things she thought she forgot. There was clarity in their priceless exchange. Her polished fingers twirled her hair pulling him in closer into her stories. Under the table, her toes raised themselves in the girlish delight of it all. Between them, her purse comfortably napped on the small table without the slightest worry of being grabbed or whisked away by traveling thieves.

After a time, Violet puffed up her hair with her hands and said, "Oh, I must go. I have so much to do. It was so nice meeting you and thank you again for catching my fall. I don't know what would have happened to me if you weren't there."

Skeeter smiled and kissed her hand, *"It was fate. We were meant to meet and be together."*

"Well, I don't know about that, but I must say it was a most enjoyable afternoon." Violet could not find a reason to leave except to possibly catch her breath. She was dizzy, confused. Perhaps it was his cologne.

"Please don't leave. What do you have to do?"

"Well... I don't…" Violet looked around the empty gymnasium for some answer. "I… I don't exactly remember at the moment what it is… but I am a very busy woman. That I know for sure. And at some point today I have to bake two trays of my special rolled cabbage horns. Everyone loves them, you know." She caught her words in flight and giggled. "Of course you don't know that. We just met."

He smiled and added an irresistible wink. There was something about this woman. He wanted to spend the entire day with her.

She discarded her excitement and his flirtatious gestures and went about the business she could not remember. Her ill-fated memories could explain nothing. Violet simply knew she needed to return to Chicago, return home to the corner back room with the tall windows that stood shoulder-to-shoulder. The neighborhood birds that sat on outside branches would wonder where she had been but Violet felt assured they would say nothing to anyone of her absence.

*

I fell asleep on the couch reading The Horse's Mouth. The book slid out from my hand, fell to the floor and shook me awake. A semi-reliable clock on the other side of the room read 3:18 AM. I must have slept for hours. Outside the cold jellied the windows.

My senses were startled but eventually calmed down and focused their attention toward my mother. She was wide-awake sitting upright in her bed. She looked beautiful, rested, untouched. Her legs bent under the covers, her toes pointed up in the air wiggling the covers. The dark fell apart around her making way for the moon to get a closer look at this tiny woman. I couldn't stop staring at her. She looked like she could lead a parade of elephants. Her face seemed to be holding a secret or no knowledge whatsoever. There was a stack of dreams between us.

Cookie, Dora and Princess Belle were suspiciously quiet.

”Mom... mom, do you want something? Do you have to go to the bathroom?”

“No.” The answer was quick like a girl with a secret.

“Do you want something to drink... maybe some Ensure?"

"No. Not really... “

Quiet.

“... but I do have a taste for some jasmine tea. That would be good. Make me a warm cup of jasmine tea?”

"Tea? Jasmine tea? Really?" This was a coffee drinking house. "We don’t have any tea. I'll have to pick some up at the grocery tomorrow. We better get some sleep for now."

I tucked the blankets around my mother and kissed her. "Good night. Sweet dreams."

*

It was 9:18 in the morning.

The room was tightly packed with the aroma of freshly brewed coffee. The pot on the counter had just finished rapidly perking itself into a frenzy and stopped. God I loved Sovina. The first thing she did every morning was start making the coffee. Strong European coffee. On working days and even on her free days before she left the house, she never missed making coffee. Today Sovina was working.

"Upsy-daisy, Mrs. Violet." With one arm behind her back and the other on her right arm, Sovina lifted Violet's back and helped her turn in place. Violet would then scoot her butt from side to side until she successfully reached the edge of the mattress. When she finished her scoot and her legs hung freely, Sovina would bend down and slip on Mrs. Violet's house slippers; the pink ones with the dotted rubber bottoms.

"Ready to start your day Mrs. Violet?" Every word from Sovina poured out like sweetened milk.

Violet stretched out her arms to Sovina and held on until her wobble rested securely on the rubber handles of her walker. Once her bones were centered for travel, Violet pushed her walker quickly *out-of-the-gate* and shuffled to the bathroom just a few yards away. Violet knew Sovina was close behind and that she would help her on the toilet.

"Slow down Mrs. Violet. I can hardly keep up with you. You move like the Gods took twenty years off your legs in the middle of the night."

Sovina followed. It was something she did most every morning. At the sink she ran warm water over a washcloth and placed it on the corner of the counter. Sometimes while waiting, Violet would dampen her restless cold hands with the warm cloth.

Sovina waited and looked into the mirror. She pulled back the loose strands of her hair behind her ear while Violet sat concentrating and squeezing her cheeks in prayer. Violet was always careful when she sat on the toilet. She was worried about splashing outside the porcelain bowl, dripping on her panties, so she used all her brains and thought very hard. Sovina stood close by and occasionally touched the chenille covered bones of Violet's shoulder for encouragement.

My legs would drag my bones up the steps and into my mother's room, before I would meet my coffee, Sovina took care of my mother's morning urinations. We grew to be close friends Sovina and I. My mother's dementia was a two+ woman job.

"Hey Sovina." I walked into the room warmly robed, my eyes tucked behind sunglasses and barely open; my hair still tangled in sleep. Traffic reports from the radio slid across the counter and fell on the carpet muffling its sound. The room was god-awful bright. The light burnt my eyes through a tiny slit in my squint. My glasses only muffled the pain.

"Morning Suzka. Your coffee just finished perking." Sovina had placed my favorite cup next to the pot on the counter.

"Hey mom, how are you doing this morning?" - words that followed me from behind my intentions.

When my mother heard my voice on this particular morning, her face changed. She quickly opened her eyes wide. They stuck in place like on a silly girl in her teens an inch away from getting caught crawling back into her bedroom window before anyone noticed she was missing in the night.

"Morning Mom." I said it louder.

She looked at me for a moment and spoke quietly... *Good morning.*

Outside the opened window, two young birds argued as they were rearranging the twigs in their nest. My legs kept moving without any orders and took me into the room's bathroom. Once there, I picked up an elongated tray setting on the toilet's tank. The girl resembling a disheveled version of myself in the bathroom's mirror tried to get my attention but I gave her little notice.

The tray was lined and arranged like an artist's palette with colors, powders and creams. The little woman yards away sitting like the grasshopper in her wheelchair, was my canvas. No woman, no painter, no canvas should start the day, any day, without color.

As I brought the tray closer to my mother, I noticed a few items missing; a few items were always missing. They were most likely snatched in the night, taken shortly after one of my mother's *under-the-radar* bathroom visits. There was no use asking the little lady. She had no credible clues and had no idea the measure of her own criminal activities. Luckily, she was a terrible thief. She always hid her stash (sometimes a tube of lipstick or blush) in the same retrievable place – the freezer, under the nut rolls.

"Did you see where the…?" I asked.

"Well that's a pretty silly question to ask me." My intended inquiry was suspiciously cut in half, chopping off the question part. Violet continued in her defense. "I never saw anything. Go next door and talk to the neighbors. They're the people you should be talking to. That's what I think. Oh Lord Jesus, if only people would be sensible and not turn to crime. I'm just lucky I caught the last bus."

I hadn’t a clue what she was talking about.

Violet was most anxious sitting in her chair. Disoriented, her hands cupped into each other as if they were holding on to a captured lightning bug from the night's play. Her head worked hard on forgetting the feelings left over from her amorous dream.

Sovina brought me my coffee.

My mother quickly snapped herself into the moment in front of her. Her voice returned to its home in her throat. "Hello... Good morning... I'm here..." she said.

"What do you mean? Of course you’re here, mom. Where else would you be?”

My mother kept a careful watch on her words. She pursed her lips tightly and wiggled a bit in her chair.

I placed the tray with the colors and brushes on her lap. She looked down at the assortment carefully scanning each unrecognized item. It was part of our morning ritual - a ritual that is repeated every day in Dementialand.

"Why... is this all for me?"

"Yea, everything on this tray, all these colorful cosmetics are for you mom."

In another world, another time, I would have taken a drag from a cigarette before beginning this process. All great artists standing before a blank canvas used tobacco to ignite creative inspiration. But that was almost ten years ago. I broke up with smoking.

"So how was your night? Did you have good dreams?" I asked.

Violet controlled her face tightly in thought. *Why did she say that? Why would she ever say that? She never cared about my dreams before. She must know, but how? How did she ever know?* Violet screamed at her eyes, their lids and her eyebrows. *Don't move. Don't look up. Stay perfectly still.* She kept her head sternly casual. Violet had to be sure not to look into this woman's eyes holding the tray of cosmetics for fear that she, this make-up painter, this funny faced strange woman in front of her who suspiciously moved into her home, might uncover her night's secret; crossing the border, her fall and her handsome admirer, Skeeter.

A sip of my coffee steamed my face. "Yes. It's going to be a good day, today. Let's start with the lipstick. Do you want lipstick? Of course you do. We need to give this day a fighting chance and arm ourselves with… *lipstick.*"

Her head stirred around the words like she was cooking a stew. "Yes, yes, lip-stig. Give me the lip-stig."

"Blush too?" I showed her the container. "Powder?"

"Yes. Give me the powder."

The canvas of my mother's skin was thin. The structure in her face stood out like an abandoned building. Mom stretched her neck and pushed her head's face out as far as it would go to meet the brush's bristles half way. Anxious powders jumped off the brush and fell to my mother's cheeks while others hung onto the hairs of the brush waiting for my direction. I spread the dust gently high into her bones.

Next to the blush's powder on the tray was a tube of red lipstick. My choice. I loved lipstick and always wore the color red. It was part of who I painted myself to be.

Before the cylinder cover left the tube, my mother squeezed her furrowed lips together and pushed them in position waiting for the polish to be applied. I pressed the creamed color against her lips and smeared it into the creases in an attempt to fill in the faded lip's outline. As I stepped back to check my work, she pressed the surface of her lips together to stamp in the color. Some things a woman does instinctively and never forgets.

"Now, the earrings Mom. Pick the pair of earrings you want to wear today."

Four pair of earrings lay on the mirrored tray. "Pick any pair you like."

She looked at the earrings carefully and touched each one with her index finger. This was a slow and careful process. "I will take this one." It was always the same. She would pick the large round clip-ons with black and gold chips in a geometric design.

"There. Now you look simply beautiful. You are ready for all the surprises life has in store for you today. Nothing can go wrong when a woman is wearing earrings and lipstick."

"You know mom, it's the Miss America Pageant tonight. Big night for gowns and glitter." Violet never missed attending the pageants in her living room for as long as I can remember.

"Wha?" Translated meant *What in God's earth are you talking about?*

"The Miss America Pageant… it's on TV tonight."

"Ohhhh." It was a sheepish response with no understanding.

"Let's see. Why don't we use the fancy clip on your hair this time, that one with the shiny rhinestones." I picked a clip that was sitting on the crippled table. It was perfect.

"You know what... of course. Wait a minute. Don't move. I'll be right back."

I ran downstairs. In a box on the pool table that held an assortment of misplaced trinkets was a crown. One of those old prom-type tiaras with backcombs that kept the crown from falling off a queen's head. I grabbed it and pulled away the chains and other baubles that stuck to the jeweled piece. Then I noticed to the side of my vision, a vase filled with plastic flowers, daisies, dusty yellow daisies. I grabbed the bunched arrangement, shook the dust off in the air and ran back up the stairs.

"Voila!" The final touch! Sovina finished brushing her hair, clipped it in place and added the crown. We presented her with the conventional arrangement of flowers, a bouquet of dusty daisies. "You are the crowned Queen of Dementialand." She looked extraordinary. I heard her giggle some words but I couldn't understand.

She held the flowers in her arms that entire day and adjusted her crown once or twice as if she were waiting for Bert Parks to walk in and start singing, *There She Is…*

*

Miles away in time, Skeeter could not get Violet off his mind. He thought of her night and day. Something about her burnt into his chest. He fell beneath the surface of his mission. A silent animal filled with anguish, filled with joy consumed him. He replayed their first meeting in his head over and over again. His thoughts were of worshipping her.

He finally called Violet and spoke in the tenderness reserved only for lovers.

"Violet, Miss Violet this is Skeeter... the gentleman you met at the border yesterday. I hope I am not being intrusive but I wanted to check on your injury and see if you have recovered fully after your fall."

"Skeeter? Skeeter from the...?" Violet looked around the room and then down at her ankle. She thought maybe he was part of a dream, a wonderful dream. The type of dream you play again in your head repeatedly when no one is looking and later thank the dream fairies for leaving it under your pillow.

"How is your ankle, Miss Violet?"

"Why... it's... It's fine. I'm fine. Where..." Violet looked down at her ankle. Puzzled. Trying so hard to put the pieces together. Her caller's voice was toying with her sense of order. She didn't like what was happening. Aside her confusion the handsome caller waited.

"You must go away. My daughter will be coming back into the room soon."

"She won't be able to hear me. I came to see you, only you."

A mosquito buzzed around her head. She waved her hand in the air to stop its pest'ing.

"Miss Violet, I would like to see you again, perhaps we can visit sometime today."

"Today? ...Today?" Violet looked around the empty room to see if anyone overheard her thinking. She went back into her head and answered her persistent pursuer.

"Are you crazy? I can't meet with you and how did you find me anyway? Where did you come from? You have to go away. Leave right now." Her head voice wasted no time in responding.

"I am so sorry if I make you nervous. I assure you my intentions are truly honest and loving."

"I am sure they are but I have a life here. With a family... I… I think I have children too… I think I have girl children." All her thoughts were bumping into each other. "Oh, don't confuse me. You're... "

"I am not here to confuse you. Quite the contrary."

"You're making no sense. Just go away... and don't take anything with you when you leave. Everything here is mine." Violet wasn't sure what she was saying. Words fell out of her mouth with no mind and no malice.

"I will only go away if you promise to meet with me. Perhaps later this afternoon."

"You must go away... someone is going to catch you... oh my God, I can't be caught talking to you. Stop talking to me and go away please."

"Not until you promise."

29.
ELLIE AND HER FATHER

Mrs. Violet was sitting in a wheelchair, sipping through a straw her butter-pecan Ensure. The balloons of Cookie, Kitty, Dora and Belle were at her side, carefully overseeing the concerns of the little lady and looking out for possible danger or harm that might come to her. Violet's eyes fixed on a strange man standing in front of her. She stared at him as she twisted her drinking straw, trying to remember if he was a man she should know; someone who perhaps was hidden in her memory's blind spot. This man for sure was not her visiting admirer, Skeeter.

Ellie came to the house for a visit. She brought sweet smelling violets, a viola alba plant and a box of almond horn cookies from a local bakery… and she brought her father. Ellie's father was about my mother's age. His wife died four years ago. Although I told my mother about Ellie and her father coming to visit, she acted surprised when they walked into the room. She watched his head curiously move around the room from one balloon to another. There were twelve that day; 'airheads' that floated with authority above all visiting guests.

The old man's eyes widened like a schoolboy at a circus. There was Dora, Elmo, Tweety-Bird, a couple of Mermaids and God only knows how many butterflies. He gave each ballooned airhead a proper amount of attention. But when he got to Dora and followed her ribbon down to the arm of Violet's wheelchair, something snapped inside his head and returned him to the old man he was.

The fatherly man bent over and extended his hand to Violet. That hand hung in the air like a buzzard flying around in a desert looking for a place to dine. I gave my mother a little nudge on her shoulder to do the polite thing and extend her hand for the shaking but under her breath she indicated, *she wouldn't* and she didn't. Eventually he pulled his arm back.

Ellie broke the ice. "Violet, this is my father. He wanted to meet you. He is visiting with my family for a couple of weeks."

"You are so pretty. My daughter never told me you were such an attractive lady."

My mother bit down on the straw and tightened her plated teeth into her gums and said nothing.

"How wonderful to finally meet you. My daughter told me so many wonderful things about you."

Violet turned her head slightly and sunk back into the chair. Under her arm, she covertly maneuvered the handles of her purse with a tight grip. I hadn't a clue what she was thinking. She adored Ellie and her father seemed nice enough, a tall man about the height of my father with white hair boxed to his head. His trousers were high. His back was bowed. Not sure if that was an impairment or an intentional gesture to get closer to my mother who was considerably lower in height.

We moved the seat-able furniture around in a circle. An ottoman was in the center where a tray with goodies and fancy napkins leaned slightly to one side.

"Here... Sit right here." I pulled out a chair for the bowed man. "Take this seat." The chair was the furthest and safest distance away from my mother.

"Would you like some coffee? And Ellie, why don't you sit next to my mom over there." I loved Ellie's visits. She always brought over a bit of positive light when she visited. It was packaged in her laugh.

Earlier I placed cups and saucers on the counter - the fancy china. Mom had seven different china sets. I selected the set that best suited our visiting guests. The cups had an ornate flower pattern with green deco trim around the lip. Its twin saucer wore the same circle. But the best part was the inside of the cup. It looked as if each cup was delicately painted in liquid pearls, the same paint God used to brush the insides of abalone shells. Ellie's father looked abalone'ian.

My mother straightened her back and stretched her neck as far as it would go. Something took over her with utmost priority. Her vision tunneled its way to the counter. The dementias had already robbed her of the peripheral parts of her room. But now her eyes were more directed and focused as if looking through a toilet paper roll.

She looked to the china pieces sitting on the counter and moved her lips in counting each cup and saucer as if the count would be needed to match the number at the end of the visit. I could see her eyes trying to memorize each piece. She would have to be right this time. She knew that if she was to forget what was stolen then nothing was ever stolen in the first place. And 'they' would have gotten away with it.

I sternly looked at her and telepathically sent her a message as loud as I could. *Pick up my words mommy dearest. Pick up my words... He's not gonna take one of your frigin' china cups. I can see what you're doing. You're not fooling anybody.* She paid me no attention.

Violet was exceptionally alert. She followed our conversation and every joke. Her eyes were wide and bright and moved from Ellie to her father to Sovina and myself.

It was somewhat surreal staying in that very moment. My mother was not my mother and I was not her middle child but someone who made her laugh often and argued with her less than anyone else. Sovina might have argued but her tone was so gentle and soft even if she did one would ever notice.

And then she spoke. Violet looked directly at Ellie's father. "How's your boil."

"What boil?"

"I heard it was a boil you had."

The man just sat there like a grilled fish on a bed of parsley. The room was quietly confused and held its air in place.

"Mom, where did you ever get that idea?"

"Someone told me he had a boil."

We all looked at Violet as if she were a riddle.

"No." Ellie gently answered. "My father doesn't have a boil. Where did you ever get that idea, Violet?"

"Well, someone told me he had a boil." Violet looked assuredly at Ellie.

My mother, for as long as I've known her had never accepted being called into question, especially if its focused intent was to prove her wrong. That rule she never lost to the dementias.

Violet sat there with an absent-minded smile given out of accomplished politeness. The words were left out of the stable now, running willy-nilly without ownership.

"Someone told me he got the boil from one of those massage places he visited?"

Oh my God. If it was of any comfort to Ellie's father, my mother had lost all the social implications pertaining to massage parlors and displayed a genuine concern toward his condition.

Ellie felt she had to say something. "You might have heard me talk about my brother Bill. He was the boy (sounds like boil) my father had from a prior marriage. But he doesn't have a boil."

"Well my dear…" Ellie's father nudged his daughter's arm to get her attention. "You know Bill's mother might have worked in a massage parlor at one time."

Violet continued. "I can just imagine how you must feel. Having such a terrible thing like a big boil. We had a dog when I was a little girl that I loved more than anything in the world. One day he ran out into the street and got hit by a car. I just didn't think I would ever get over it."

[Gradually my mother's body was stuck
only to the facts she created at that moment.
Everything else was understandably…

unreasonable.]

We sat there dumbfounded watching our afternoon conversation being slaughtered. The balloons nervously bumped into each other. Dora spoke, *"What is girlfriend talking about? Someone rescue this little darling from herself."*

I was hoping Ellie's father would just stop talking to my mother, but he didn't. "I'm sorry about your dog. I also have very great love for animals and children too." He was so sympathetic that I wanted to jump out of my skin. He went on moving his lips and then I saw they were moving by themselves, like a preacher.

My mother was armed. "And are you declaring yourself to having a saintly nature?"

"Oh no… I don't think I... well I never gave that much thought..."

"You look saintly."

I found myself lunging out of my chair. I picked up the tray of almond horns, secretly begging the powdered cookies to help in changing the subject. "We also have mom's cabbage horns that I just thawed out this morning. You love my mother's cabbage horns don't you?" Ellie and Sovina regained their senses adding "Oh yes, Violet's cabbage horns. We love them. Thank you. That would be great." Sovina jumped up first and moved quickly to the counter where the thawed horns sat as backup.

Ellie's father didn't like talking about boils or dead dogs but had the sense about him to change the subject.

"Look at that bird over there on the lawn. It has golden eyes. Can you see him Violet? …over there. Can you see his eyes? That is a Barrow's Goldeneye."

"No, I think you're wrong... I am sure that's a duck."

Violet squinted forward in her chair, moving a slight bit closer to the window; a gesture she thought would show more scientific clarification and back up her sighting.

"Yes, I'm sure that's a duck." Those were fighting words.

She looked as if she used up all her conversation skills. From that point on, the afternoon took on all the qualities of a bad dream, lurid and grotesque. At times my mother's naïveté made her words skip around like a young lamb, equivalent to a genius who had overcome the conventional boundaries of fact. Yet its bizarre intensity had a kind quality of demented splendor.

I began to feel a strong sense of tranquility as I sat there watching her face. How distant she seemed, separated by the shadows and panes of the sunlight that fell between the trees. I must have murmured something or sighed, for she turned to look at me and softly asked, "Do I know you?"

Slowly, Violet ventured out of all conversations. She would drop her head, rest her thoughts someplace that she would later forget and stare out on the lawn. She did not speak for some time.

Before the old man left the room, he bent over and kissed my mother on the cheek. *Oh my God...* I softly whispered to myself… *this is NOT going to be good.*

"It was a pleasure meeting you Violet and I do hope we can get together again while my stay in Chicago."

As the door closed behind them, before Ellie and her father left the stoop, my mother jumped out of her chair. She raised her shaking fingers and held them in the air like the hands of the angels in church. "Did you see that? Did you see what he did?" She gave me a look as if she wanted to poison me. "I swear on the grave of all the saints in heaven, there is no way I am going to marry that man and take care of all his kids... and his boil too! I am as free as a bird right now - I have my own life... I have a sec-terry..."

Violet sat back into her chair. The storm inside her had passed.

She pulled down her skirt to readjust its covering over her knees. Calmly she looked at her hands, pressing down the wrinkles on the skirt's pattern; tiny horn shapes resembling the cookies she made with her mother and that she made with her children, although she did not remember. They were locked in an empty space inside, where a small girl's hands rolled almond horns in powered sugar and placed them on a shiny oiled baking sheet. Horn shaped cookies baked and wrapped in wrinkled wax paper were tied with string and placed in the side pocket of her purse where the other wrapped memories were hidden.

Sovina and I cleared the dishes and shared a cold Saris beer.

The day could only fold itself shut in its own time.

*

"Violet. Miss Violet."

Violet recognized the voice and knew what she had promised. It was Skeeter. She looked around the room. Suzka and Sovina were busy at the counter drinking their beer. She ignored his call at first.

"Violet. Miss. Violet, it's Skeeter. Remember?"

Violet looked around the room twice and turned her head to the window as to redirect the landing of her words. Hopefully the window curtains would swallow the sound before they could be heard in the room.

"I'm busy now. Go away."

"I'm not going away. You know why I'm here Miss Violet. You promised."

"Oh... I know... " Desperately Violet tried to remember the certain amount of excuses she had prepared. "But this is not a good time. I will meet you later... you know... later, the much, much later time... when it's dark, yes in the nighttime, you know. I promise. Just, just go away before someone walks in."

"I will come back for you after the sun is down and the night is dizzy."

"Oh no, no. That will never work. Where's my remote? I have MetLife... I am dead sure I have MeLife at that time."

Violet dare not move save for the tiniest quiver of her lips. "You are so confusing me."

"I will see you tonight, Miss Violet; after your work is done."

Violet tightly held her smile and took a deep breath sucking in her secret. She closed her eyes and raised her shoulders. Something changed inside of her. She heard her soft voice surrender in girlish excitement... 'He called'.

Birds outside stopped what they were doing and shook their heads.

[It was about that time when
I began calling my studio
leaving long messages on my
answering machine. I needed
a part of me to be in my studio
– even if it was just my voice.]

Later that night, Violet sat in her chair, unbuttoned the thin silk button of her bed jacket and waited.

She looked around the empty room checking if there was anyone close who could possibly hear conversations she would have with Skeeter; if he actually would appear for their visit. There was no guarantee. This could all be a terrible trick.

She twiddled her mind in distraction and began rehearsing the numerous excuses she would use if Skeeter did return. Violet was determined to take better control over her new beau's demands. She would be direct and say words like... *'Maybe tomorrow. I'm busy today,'* or *'I think that girl, the one with the painted shoes is taking me somewhere'.* Or possibly she thought, she should be more forceful, threaten with – *'The police are here... The house is on fire!' No, no, no, that won't work,'*

Violet lined up her excuses and hoped she would not forget their order. *'Remember he will have a certain amount of excuses on his own. Don't let him get on your nerves'*, she told herself.

Violet knew she was forgetting things. Somewhere, there was a young man she met and married. It was a picture floating under water. She tried to remember. She would watch it disappear and reappear in the water.

"Miss Violet. It is Skeeter."

Once he spoke her name, once she heard his call in that seductive deep tone, all the excuses in her head blew away like feathers on a dandelion that had lost its voice. How could anyone resist the passionate desires from such an ardent fiery man? Where was her Jesus?

"Hello Miss Violet. It is an absolutely beautiful night. The Gods of all the worlds created this night just for you."

Violet heard his voice but did not answer. She was filled with serious confusion.

Remembering he had a certain amount of persuasion and a double rapture. Keep cool, she thought.

"Are you ready? I have wonderful plans for us. You must come. I will not take no for an answer. The sky has already turned on its stars for our arrival."

Violet looked around. She thought she saw two birds on the opposite side of the window watching but they were asleep in their nests. Violet was alone and defenseless.

"Well, I don't know... "

She tilted her head to one side and sternly whispered to Skeeter under her skin.

"You are truly acting like a crazy man. You think I can just pick-up leave here at any time. I hardly know you. Yes we met and talked a bit a few days ago… I can't remember exactly when it was but... anyway, everyone is going to get suspicious. They would think me insane if they knew I ran off with some strange handsome man in the middle of the night. They would send me away for sure."

The time assigned for respectable decision-making was scrambled and soon would be completely ignored.

Violet was tangled in thoughts. What was she ever going to do? How could she fight the dementias? She held on to her purse tightly – the purse filled with everything that held her in place – all the memories she couldn't remember. Both hands gripped the purse's straps. Even if she said no, he would surely come back. The dementias deranged all thoughts of decency.

If she only knew specifically the times Skeeter would call for her, when he wanted her. If she could somehow know in advance of his visits, the gaping disruptions with his exotic escapades, possibly then she could box them in short meetings throughout the day as not to be noticed.

Violet, like a stuffed doll floating down stream had a marvelous secret just under her skin.

Skeeter waited for her as she hid behind the veil of white purity and camouflaged memories. He didn't care how she came to him or the battles she fought with meningitis and encephalitis that rearranged her brain. He simply wanted to be with her. He was in love, completely, utterly in love with this tiny woman.

Skeeter's smile softened his words. *"No one will think you insane. You are too clever for that. We will be very careful. Trust me. Just slip on your red sequined gown and say you will go with me. We will laugh, dance and party 'till dawn. You will be very happy, trust me."*

Violet stood at a locked gate. Skeeter handed her a key and pointed to the gate's door, the door that would lead her to everything. Her curiosity cautiously hoped she would squeeze through.

On the other side, a tall handsome man carried a tiny bouquet of daisies and a larger than life father turned his head and winked at Violet to come. Birthday parties and family dinners were everywhere, people danced in step, singers sung in tune. Prairies of plastic flowers came to life spraying the air with their desired scent. There she would remember everything - everything she created.

*

In time, Skeeter grew more ruthless and demanding as their love grew. His frayed patience tore at his heart and pressed hard against his chest. If she would not come to him, he had no choice but to take her without permission, just short of rape. He would have to grab her by the shoulders and shake her, ripping open her silk and exposing her breasts. Pearl buttons that once buttoned down her memories would fall to the ground and roll away.

30.
ESPIONAGE AND OTHER SUSPECIOUS ACTIVITIES

The house was strangely quiet. The muses were asleep and the moon was quite full that particular night.

I was downstairs trying to sleep but the sheets on the leather couch made my dreams slip and slide out of my head. Maybe popcorn would convince my dreamy delusions in coming back. I rolled off the leather and made my way up the stairs. The hum of the heater was loud from moving the heavy air out of my way. Twice its forced air slapped me in the face before I got to my mother's room. The room was covered in moonlight muting the furnishings' hard edges.

At first I couldn't find my mother. The couch was neatly dressed and empty. The sheet was folded proper-like and the blanket appeared not to have a clue of my mother's whereabouts. Her purse was peeking out from under the couch's pillow.

Behind the sofa was my mother - vertically awake and seemingly on a mission. I questioned my eyes. This tiny woman stood ironed flat against the windowed wall and positioned like a jumper on the narrow ledge of a twenty-storied building. Her hands were pressed back and at her side; one hand gripped the lace drapes, the other hand held the remote control. Mom stood unbent which caused her height to exceed its five-foot stature.

I watched her from the other side of the room. The moon chalk-lined her exact location. I squinted my eyes and moved them closer into my mother. From where I was standing, I could see that she was wearing a satin pink bed jacket over her day clothes. A part of the dress she was wearing earlier stuck out of the jacket's collar. On her head, bunched hairs were claw-clipped in scattered places. A few hairs tried to escape but were captured by her large round clip-on earrings. Mom never ever went anyplace without her earrings.

My mother then scooted on the jumper's ledge and shuffled her way to the far end of the curtains. When she reached the corner, she split the curtains with the barrel of her remote control, which allowed only one eye to peek though.

The room was eerie quiet. The moon had whispered my presence into my mother's ear. She turned her head startled at first but unrelenting. I must have felt like a hunter pointing a loaded rifle at a mother dear. She kept a guarded distance and visually interrogated my intentions.

"Shhhhh" pressing the edge of the remote to her lips.

What is she doing? I raised both my eyebrows and lowered my head a tiny bit looking straight into her eyes - a gesture requesting some direction, some answers. I am not completely sure but I believe at that very moment dementia took mercy on the little woman and squeezed out a few flashbacks of a rebellious middle child that solidified her decision to trust me.

"I'm glad you're here. You can help me."

I felt strangely close to my mother, mischievous and a bit dirty. We were a team, partners in a crime. We were

Thelma and Louise, Cheech-n-Chong, the *Easy Riders* of the moment. I moved closer to the little commander for instructions.

"Now watch carefully. Watch very, very carefully. They're out there, hiding behind those trees, waiting. Can you see them?" Without Violet moving her eyes from the window, she continued updating me on the facts.

"They get their boys to do all the work. They're big boys and strong too. They come out late at night when they think I'm in sleep. And that's when they start stealing my land."

Violet quickly looked toward me and pumped up her seriousness. "They've done this before."

It appeared to me that my mother was not yet comfortable with her liberating dementias. She didn't trust their gifts of freedom or the ageless voice inside her soul. What more would she have to give to the dementias to stay in their good graces? They fed on memories - memories she was not willing to give up, not without good reason. She would remain fooling everyone, keep her screams muted and bite down on God's graces. She kept her thoughts suspicious. Paranoia just laughed and threw in all kinds of scenarios to keep Violet distracted.

I had to be very careful with my questions. I was walking a thin line. "How do they steal your land?"

"You know how they do it?" Violet obviously turned her ears off and never heard my question. But I was sure she felt my interest to be sincere.

"They move it. See those stones? They move all those stones one foot over onto my property." The accused stones were stacked like a hedge about three feet high and two feet wide extending the full length of the property. They sat precisely on the property line of the two lots for decades. The stoned hedge was in Violet's full view from the room's line of windows. The only thing between Violet and the stones was the garden of plastic begonias.

Violet lowered her voice. "That's what they do when I'm not looking… one stone at a time."

Violet retreated from her rigid surveillance and added arm gestures and twisted body animations to strengthen her argument. "In the middle of the night they move all those stones over a foot into my yard. They do it carefully so I don't notice. Then when I get up in the morning my yard is smaller. That's how they steal my land. They're sly." She repeated it again. "They take a foot at a time."

Violet finished relating the facts and returned her attention to the alleged crime scene. It was tensely quiet. The hum of the heater lowered its voice. We all waited.

"This is a criminal of fence in the sight of God and the church. And it's a sin too. A Goddam moral sin... a morbid sin... or mortal, well, you know what I'm talkin' bout… one of those big ones. I can't remember all those sins they have now. We got so many it's hard to remember all of 'em."

Violet paused. Her words were pacing back and forth in her head and gaining momentum. "They think I'm stupid just because I'm old. They think I don't know what they're doing. Well I sure as hell do. And now I am going to catch them in the act. Then you and I can... well, we'll call somebody… we'll call the land officials and we'll call the police. We can call Joe Novatny! Yes, Joe has a lot of connections. He knows people. You remember Joe don't you?"

[Joe was a policeman and friend to my father.
When I was picked up for driving without a license,
hitting a tree and another car after running a stop sign
and put in a holding cell… my father called Joe.]

"Everyone is gonna know what they're up to. I got'em this time."

Violet's words screamed to a halt. The sound was like teeth on ice. Her eyes opened, her eyes closed. She squeezed her madness out, madness so black it seemed purple. The moon was agitated, shining so fiercely it dared any cloud to get in its way.

I knew the more Violet talked the angrier she would get. And I knew that if I tried to convince her otherwise, all hell would break loose.

I was not about to question my partner's credibility.

"I'm here with you. We'll catch'em. Just tell me what to do." I slowly moved in closer to the wall and put my body in the surveillance position. A blue soft light hunched over both of us, a kind gesture from the moon that he joined our mission.

"Don't let them see you, shhhhhh, talk quietly. They don't know we're watching."

I slowly leaned over and quietly asked a question like a good partner. "What do these boys look like? I mean how big are these neighbor boys?"

"I said big, for cryin' out loud. You know... BIG. Don't you know anything? What's the matter with you?" Her voice was despairingly agitated. "Shush now." Violet did not fully trust my intentions. She must have felt she had no choice but to give me a meaningless task. "You just watch my purse," pointing to the stuffed black bag partially covered by the couch's pillow. "Keep an eye on it so no one steals it."

The situation was tenuous. Violet was unsteady. She wasn't sure where the enemy lines were drawn and who to trust. For now she would have to keep one eye on the neighbors and the other on my intentions.

"I don't know who you are but if you're NOT going to help, just get otta' here."

"I'm sorry. Like I said, just tell me what you want me to do."

Everyone was quiet.

The airheads in the room barely moved in fear of squeaking against each other.

The trees' leaves turned to look, the tenant birds peeked over the edges of their nests. On the ground, the plastic begonias tried to focus their attention but they either couldn't see what was going on or they simply didn't want to be part of my mother's paranoia. Violet stopped talking. Everything was mute. Time just sat in the moon's night waiting for instructions, waiting for something to happen.

"Mom, I'm hungry. Do you have any ice cream?"

The sound of ice cream seemed to slap the damp air out the room. The modus operandi had changed. From that razor edge moment, my mother changed her tone like a commercial in the middle of a TV crime drama. It was as if she pressed the pause button on her remote. Her voice softened the room and the world of reconnaissance.

"I love ice cream!" she said in a perky warm voice.

We shuffled our way into the kitchen, side-by-side, moving hand-in-hand as if we were glued together. The room's large windows went with us. When we got close to the refrigerated destination we stopped.

Together we slid down into a squat and pressed our backs against the cabinet doors just under the counter top. It was a safe place where we could not be seen. Then all at once I went for the Kenmore's handle.

"The light, the light, they'll see..." Violet still had a few remnants of paranoia in her head.

The refrigerator's breath steamed out. Before Violet could finish talking, I frantically grabbed the only container I could see, hoping it was ice cream, hoping it was butter pecan and slammed the door quickly. Not sure who was playing with whom at this point for I actually started to enjoy my part in her dementia. It was full of excitement and quite freeing.

I opened a drawer above my head and let my hand rummage through the utensil tray for two spoons. Despite it being quite dark, I took a quick look at the outside of the frozen carton. For sure it was ice cream. I thought myself to be lucky at that point and opened the top lid of the winning butter pecan.

“It’s butter pecan, mom. Your favorite.” and handed her a spoon.

"Oh dearie, we can't eat ice cream out of the carton. We need bowls. Open that cupboard over there.” She pointed to the lower cabinet door just a few feet away.

“Let's use the fancy Bavarian bowls with the scalloped trim and tiny pink and yellow roses. They’re on the second shelf in the back. The flowers are hand-painted, you know. Margie bought that set for me when she lived on Harlem Avenue. It was our ten, no maybe it was our fifteenth wedding anniversary...”

I turned my head and looked at this stranger, previously my mother, as if she was an alien from some other planet; an alien who also had a sister named Margie. *Where did all this recovered memory come from?*

I couldn’t move. You would have thought I was a Rodin’s sculpture commemorating the experience. Her story about the china kept going on and on, falling all over the place and landing on top of me. *How could she remember that?* Not only knowing precisely where the bowls were located in the kitchen but their damn history for God’s sake.

It might appear that this clarity could open a door for other flashes of recall but I wasn’t about to take a chance by asking her if she remembered that I was her daughter. I loved more the ambiguity of our relationship.

I pushed aside any diagnoses or medical theories and scooped two big mounds of the butter pecan into the bowl and handed it to my mother. Somewhere in that cold, creamy substance, the thieving neighbors and their nighttime activities were aborted for the night.

[Familiar memories rely more
on the brain's cortex, its outer layer,
while short-term memories rely more
on a structure called the hippocampus.
The hippocampus is typically affected
at the start of late-life dementias.]

We finished the butter pecan, got up and placed the sticky bowls on the counter. I decided to make coffee as Violet calmly walked back to the sofa. She sat down on its edge and pointed the remote control to the television while pressing down on the red button. The room filled with a bright iridescent light, the kind of light you would expect from a tiny space ship if it landed in your living room.

"Oh good, MetLife is on."

"Matlock, Mom. It's Matlock not MetLife." I tried to never correct my mother or the dementias but the MetLife-Matlock thing was making me crazy.

31.
BILLY THE VISITING NURSE

A nurse's aide came to the house twice a week. She took the vitals, chatted a bit and wrote long cursive messages on a thick yellow pad. Her notes curled their edges.

POINT OF REFERENCE

[Visiting Nurses provide services to homed patients. They monitor vital signs, such as blood pressure, heart rate, temperature and report to the doctor the patient's status and any health changes.]

"How yaw doin' today Miss Violet? Do you 'member who I am and why I'm heah?"

The aide was a woman in her mid-thirties who recently moved to Chicago from Dallas. She had a heavy accent and a heavy smile to match, both overdone like a full bottle of cheap cologne on a used car salesman, cologne that tickled Violet's nose and made her squish her nostrils shut. The aide's eyes jumped from place to place looking for land mines to extinguish. She appeared professionally plump and armed. An official identification badge with the name 'Billy' was clipped to the collar of her white coat. Under the coat Billy wore a cotton blue surgical top with matching pressed blue pants. Her shoes were whitewashed of all color. She carried with her a black case stuffed with papers ripe to escape from their folders. Violet's folder was in there someplace.

My mother was nervous that day. She had the full jitters. Her feet were particularly loud and unruly. They moved around like rowdy hooligans arguing on the front porch of her wheelchair. And her fingers pounded out the William Tell Overture around her legs as if there was an ivory keyboard sitting on her lap and tucked under her thighs. Her purse bounced in the back row. Memories that were jammed loosely in the side pouches, slid out of their order.

"Miss Violet...Miss Violet, How yaw doin' today? Do you 'member who I am and why I'm vis'tin yaw?"

I hated when people who knew my mother, who visited often, started their conversations with fixed smiles and a 'who-am-I' series of questions. I thought it condescending. Those were questions clinically reserved for halfwits walking around the cuckoo-nests in bleak institutions.

"*I second that.*" said Kitty.

All the airheads waved in agreement. Seven or maybe there were eight that day in full view behind my mother. A reasonable amount I thought to validate some attention. *Look up for God's sake.* I wanted to scream… *Look up.*

"How yaw doin' today Miss Violet? It's a beautiful day. Do you 'member who I am? Do you know wha' day 'tis? Talk to me darling, who – is – the – president? Do you know?"

I watched my mother's unresponsive attitude sink. She squirmed around and moved closer back into her wheelchair. The jitters tempted her to slip away into an empty hiding place where she could stand tippy-toed on her dementias and lasso herself to the moons and stars in the sky. I watched her temporarily disappear and thought of my mother flying away to exotic places until plump arms coming from oceans away, pulled her back into the room.

I tightened my jaw and bit down hard to stop any regretting words from slipping out. My mouth was stuffed with some of the greatest pungent, sarcastic lines that in different circumstances would have been applauded, Emmy'ed, Oscar'ed or maybe even Cleo'ed in a more appropriate and accepting setting - a gift I inherited from my father.

Dora, Betty and the Elmo twins caught in the draft, leaned over as if they were trying to help my mother. "*She's fine, you're Billy and it's a weekday - not sure which one but we got mail and Judge Judy just finished slapping around some poor schmuck's defense because he spoke while the judge's mouth was still moving. She only does that on weekdays.*"

Billy couldn't wait for Violet's answer.

She was pudgy with nursing book knowledge she learned in Dallas. All kinds of diagnoses jammed up inside of her, ready to nose-dive off her tongue.

Looking past my mother and toward me, she left her friendly self and jumped straight into her medical-ness.

"Looks like she'z got a bit of agitation in'er today and she'z not respondin' to simple queschuns."

You mean stupid questions...I thought.

Billy was excited about her prognosis and equally proud of her diagnostic and her nursie-protected opinion. She stuffed her papers and her medical-ness into her briefcase and reapplied her smile.

The visit ended.

"I'll give the doctors my repor'. They'll send'ya a prescripshun over to the house. It'll keep her quiet and calm'er down. I'll check in with ya'll tomorra."

Billy had a tailored rigid adherence to all the medical guidelines. In her visits, she offered no fresh illusions to a medical establishment that supplied more pills and clichés than answers. Like a good soldier, she fought off all invasions of external suggestions. I eventually crossed the conventional boundaries of papered prescriptions and declare war on this southern little lady. It was inevitable. Maybe not today, but it was coming.

I was uncomfortable, uneasy with most drug medications. Papered prescriptions overriding other papered prescriptions. Drugs followed by other drugs for the side effects, followed by more drugs needed to repair the damage from taking drugs. Violet was not good with most medications. No one in the family had much of a tolerance to drugs. We had our own medical concoctions and recipes for curing everything bad.

Billy ended her visit and stood over my mother. "Good – bye – Violet." A change in her tone and direction, she addressed me... "I'll check in with ya'll tomorra." Final head turn back to Violet. "Now – you – be – good – an – stay – otta' – trouble."

*

I was protective of my mother. But maybe in truth, I was defending my own forgetful ways and craziness. I loved crazy. All artists love crazy - painters for sure. Crazy smears itself on thirsty canvases hungry for involvement with the beautiful, the brilliant and the unattainable. Crazy talks to me on buses and loosens old thoughts that had been stuck in my head for years. Crazy slaps my thinking silly, wakes me up and more than often, pries opens my closed eyes. They are my ah-ha moments - those times when the gods had turned my head 180 degrees and inside out to look at life differently.

Between reality and fantasy, past and present, the palpable and the mysterious, I found living with my mother, with the dementias and the crazies, the gypsies and the saints, the airheads and the unknown, rather enjoyable in a crazy way.

*

Violet glanced sideways out of her eyes at the moon's sun. She watched its line of light under the blinds. When she thought the moon was tired, her eyes would close inside themselves like a shutter in a camera about to take a picture. Waiting.

Skeeter did come back that night and returned nearly every night after that. He found a way to crawl into

Violet's head and lure her away like a lovesick schoolboy taunting his sweetheart in meeting him outside her bedroom window.

Good evening my sweet Violet. I know this is short notice but I want you to come with me to a party. Everyone you cannot remember will be there. You must come. I will not take 'no' for an answer.

Violet tried to play the game of resistance and teased her new lover in defense of surrendering everything to him. She twirled around on unframed memories as she seductively danced for him and for everyone.

Skeeter's boyishness unlocked a hunger inside of her. Their secret affair pulled Violet closer into herself.

They talked and laughed through the night and traveled through time. He took her everywhere and danced with her in the mirror of gods and goddesses. He lavished her with gifts of silk and blest moonstones loosely strung on fine linen threads.

*

A skinny man from Walgreens stood outside the front door. He pushed his eyes closer into a side window looking for any signs of life. When he saw me on the other side, he raised the small white bag up to his shoulders and shook it back and forth, up and down like a baby's rattle.

The Calvary was here to save the jitters.

I opened the door. The temperature dropped 40 degrees. I signed for the rattling Calvary and led the bag with the pills to Dementialand, specifically to the counter where the other medical prescriptions argued with each other. The over-the-counter meds stacked themselves neatly armed for battle.

On the wall above the counter, a worn picture hung. The wedding couple inside the frame stared out at their future. They did not see a Suzka, a Sovina nor any gypsies, airheads or saints. They held their eyes still. Their clothes remained forever buttoned. A white bouquet of Calla Lilies released tiny fragrances to only the dreamers and believers that happened to pass by the framed picture.

32.
DEMENTIA'S NIGHTTIME DEMONS

It was close to midnight. It hadn't been a very good day, which left no reason for me to expect the night to be any better. Everything was off. In its morning, the sun was late and came rushing in, barely squeezing into the day before the night closed its door. Billy's visit sat in my head like bad cheese in a bad dream fouling my sleep. Sovina was upstairs with my mother.

The night screamed from above and woke me. I walked up the steps to check on my mother. The sundowning gypsies danced around her bed like they do every night but tonight the air for dancing was fast and cunningly vicious.

The airheads with their black eyes and painted smiles, squeezed against each other as if they feared being slashed to inflation. They fluttered and scooted into a huddle. All the saints of Michael and Christopher throughout the house wiggled out of their statue'ness and rushed into Violet's room for battle.

Something was horribly wrong.

"Oh my God Sovina... what's happening? Why is mom acting like that?"

My mother looked mad in her craziness. Her feet scratched the sheets like the desperate feet of trapped chickens.

"Mrs. Violet is very nervous. I've never seen her this upset."

"What brought this on?"

"I... I think it could be those new pills Billy sent over. The ones to calm her fidgetiness and help her to sleep."

She swayed her body from side to side and shook her head hard trying to push out the induced hallucinations from her head. Her face squished and distorted its fleshy-waxed skin in some clamoring determination as she moaned and mumbled absurdities.

Sovina wiped Violet's head with a cold damp rag. The room sweated with worry for my mother. I saw patches of her skull gleaming like the inside of an oyster shell. Buttons slipped open on her bed jacket in the struggle.

"Jesus. How many of those pills did she take?"

"Just two. Exactly what it said on the bottle. Only two, I swear."

My mother grabbed the rails on the side of her bed with both hands and held on tightly. Her body jerked back and forth. Her grip was secure. She grunted and tightened her thighs together. An odor stuffed the room; battleground sweat and adrenalin.

Someone took over my mother. Some THING filled the room.

I ran around useless shutting the windows with no reason in my head as to why.

Sovina cradled my mother's shoulders as a mother would when her baby had a bad dream. She stroked my mother's head and talked softly calling "Miss Violet... Miss Violet wake up. Please wake up. You are safe. No one is going to hurt you."

It was as if a chilling and diabolical visitor came into our night and filled the room.

The moon peeked through the slits of the dark sky. When it got a glimpse of our hideous visitor, its face cringed and ran behind the closest night cloud.

The visitor, a slimy creature, who was muscular and pockmarked crawled into Dementialand leaving a spittle-like trail behind. His eyes were sunken and red. His lipless mouth slobbering in excitement was lined with serrated sharp teeth that were evenly spaced in his gums.

He crawled around under my mother's bed enjoying the moment as if he was a parading tribute to everything macabre and terrifying. Like the scoundrel he was, he cursed the moment in gratefulness, in prayer, giving thanks to confused gods and mockingly laughed at the sainted patrons who came to help.

When he finished posturing himself, he tightened his claws and tore into my mother splitting her in two. He ripped out her spirit and dragged her into the murky depths, through the sagas and shanties where the descendants of some of the worst sinners lived.

This creature was not kind to his frail host and there simply was not enough room inside of my mother's tiny frame to battle it out with such a gruesome demon.

Moaning, then mumbling and finally screaming, Violet gripped the guardrail on her bed. Her hands clenched tightly around the metal. Blue bulbous veins of knotting blood mapped highways on her skin that stretched themselves as far as they could. She banged her head against the rail again and again and again with such force she could not be held back. Her face squished. Her lips pushed forward pulling the loose skin forward like a balloon deflating its air. Her eyes were hidden behind tightly closed lids. Wordless anger.

The gypsies and the saints could not help her. They were overpowered. Skeeter was nowhere in sight. He was reviving old memory trinkets, gifts he would give to Violet later that night. The ballooned heads with the painted smiles could only watch. A devil who got tired of hell came into my mother for play, menacing with her for the sport, the merriment of the moment.

Violet was forced to host this demon. He took her everywhere and nowhere. She desperately screamed for a way back, a way out, yelling for God to help.

She clamped her hands tighter to the bed rail with the sweaty strength of a prizefighter, banging her head repeatedly against the bed's rail. There was no way I was able to open her grip. Sovina held my mother's head back but Violet's agitation and strength grew. The force inside this tiny woman overpowered us. A woman with a body so small it was like a pigeon. How was this possible?

I wrapped towels around the guardrail and duct taped them in place, hoping to prevent any physical injury that my mother would do to herself. Sovina and I had no choice but to wait out the storm, to wait for the demon to leave. Calling the hospital, the hospital calling the doctor, the doctor calling Walgreens, Walgreens delivering more pills that brought more demons was not an option.

After a time, the gypsies' colors returned to their forms and the Michaels and Christophers retreated back to their places of statue. The whole room spun slower and slower. Two airheads lost some air and fainted behind the couch.

'R' give me an 'R'.

Violet fell into a damp deep sleep. The maven demon would have to wait until she woke up before he could begin tormenting her again. Demon work is exhausting. He slithered back into his plastic cylinder with its childproof cap and talked of his accomplishments with the other rival mediators. He felt pride in himself as though he was the last one standing in a bloody street massacre. Louder and louder he laughed and married himself to the other disdainful arrogant killers in the world. Killers who stood on the dead caucuses of their blindsided prey, their undermanned, unarmed, unequal opponents – victims of the demon's sport.

I'm sorry, there is no 'R'.

*

Throughout the night, I heard her call out, talking to Pavel, Andrew, Gustie, Philomena and Adeline, visitors from the Mary Queen of Heaven cemetery. Very quietly I tiptoed to her bed. She was asleep, lying with her hands curled up into fists of fear. The moonlight returned and covered her, casting a rim of radiance on her strands of hair. I kissed her cheek and whispered, "It's ok mom, everyone is here. Nothing bad is going to happen to you."

33.
THANKSGIVING

It was a cool fall day. I looked at my mother trying to make out if she knew anything – what a day it was, what was missing on this day than from the years past. There wasn't the traditional smell of turkey basting in its juices, marinating the ripe air that was hardened by our family fighting. Fighting always preceded the guests' arrival – relative guests that would later come armed with their own overcooked opinions for battle. Yet, she looked at me as if she knew I had something different planned for the day. This Thanksgiving we would have lunch at Crystal's, a Bohemian restaurant, a forgotten favorite.

The sky was as muted and grey as tap water. Violet hadn't ventured out of her room for what seemed to be months. But I convinced myself this would be a good outing for us all.

"Mom, Sovina and I were thinking about going out today and eating lunch at Crystal's. Do you want to come along? Stephan is going to meet us there. You want to come?" I always gave her the feeling that she had a choice.

She laughed with delightful approval, without a clue why.

*

The lobby at Crystal's was filled with a sea of heads colorfully covered in patterned babushkas, rain bonnets, lacquered bouffants and matted toupees that held on more to a lonely promise than improving appearances. The heads were attached to the loyal patrons of the infamous west side Bohemian restaurant.

The man-heads appeared to be less aggressive in this setting, unlike their counter parts. Their job was to squeeze their way to the front counter in order to get a numbered plastic card from the hostess. The card would confirm their place in order.

Their wives were the true warriors. They were predatory creatures that prowled around the packed lobby like hungry coyotes looking for a place to sit. Crystal's was a popular restaurant among all the locals with ties to central Europe. The wait was always long; seating was scarce.

These women warriors walked through the crowd looking at the cards held by other seated patrons. The lowest number would be leaving their chair first. Like coyotes, they were quick in their hunt. They would snatch the warm seat from a rising patron before the stamped form of their butt left its vinyl covering.

I wheeled my mother into the lobby and without second thought I desperately sought out the hostess. Hopefully it would be Elenka. She knew my mother for years. I tried to maintain a level of composure in my search but began to question my decision. I kept myself emotionally detached and intact fearing that if I didn't, all hell would break loose. There was a chance this crowd could take her to places in her head that would turn this afternoon lunch into a holocaust. This part of the process had to run smoothly.

"44"

Ah yes, Elenka! I stretched my neck into the air as far as it would go and balanced my full weight on all my toes. *Elenka, Elenka, Can you see me? I have Violet here with me. I am her daughter from California. Remember Violet?* Thoughts that screamed out into the room were noticed.

Elenka saw me. She remembered. She waved above the crowd, directing us to move forward, ahead of the 44, to the dining room area.

"Why. hello Mrs. Violet. I haven't seen you for a long time." She leaned over and kissed my mother on both cheeks. "We missed you. I have a special table just for you. Follow me."

Behind me were mumbling complaints. "Hey, we were here first? …I couldn't hear. When did they call 40?

...They can't just butt in like that. Who'd they think they are? ...I saw them come in. They're cheaters."

I turned around and said to the crowd in a sincere attempt to prevent a mob scene, "Number 24, she said 24. See..." and flashed some bogus card in the air covering the numbers with my fingers. I didn't want to get mugged in the bathroom or in the parking lot on out way out. Tough crowd.

We followed the hostess. "Your brother Stephan arrived just five minutes ago and is saving a place for you at the table by the fireplace." My mother always remembered the presence of Stephan.

The dining area was tight. There were about fifty closely placed tables with linen tablecloths under white butcher blocked paper used for the gravy's overspill. Four or maybe five heavy wood breakfronts showcased sparkling crystal glassware behind beveled glass making the room feel very European. All the windows were large and covered with lace curtains that distorted the buses, cabbies and dirtied salted cars on the other side. Snow that survived numerous falls piled itself on the curb's fringes looking grey and hardened in stubbornness.

All the servers dressed the same, short red skirts with embroidered flower appliqués, tight black corseted vests and puffed sleeved blouses. Red, yellow and gold moved quickly between the tables. The servers spoke with heavy accents. Jumbled words and dialects from two continents were mixed in the warm porcelain bowls with dimpled dumplings waiting to be soaked in gravy. Airborne trays balanced the Schnitzels, the Goulash and the Spaetzles

I looked at my mother. She was not part of any conversation at the table and did not show the least bit of interest in anything around her. She had hardly talked in the past month. Words lost their way. How damn frustrating it must be, I thought. We all need to communicate in some way, to be heard and understood, to tell people who we are. But once I moved outside myself, I noticed Violet spoke eloquently with her simple gestures, her eyes and her body. She made incredible sounds when she didn't speak.

I sat across the table from my mother. Both her hands were hidden under the linen. Her eyes sought out the blank holes in my face. I stared back, determined at first and at the same time, questionably cautious.

Her face was striking, not handsome or beautiful, it was different, lined and abandoned. She shared her smile with a kind and unpronounced gentleness. But it was in her eyes that she did all her bidding. They had a bright almost sharp clarity that brought a sense of significance to things.

She winked at me. For some stupid reason I looked around me as if her wink was intended for someone else. Then she winked again, a clear strong wink. Maybe it was her way of reminding me of the secret we shared. I really didn't know of its intention. It seems a bit silly now when I think about it but at that time I had believed she was thanking me for defending her strange behavior and protecting her craziness from being unfavorably interpreted.

She closed both her eyes and then opened them quickly. They were set, fixed and steady. There was a kind of charm about her that was very compelling. This time she raised her eyes and winked again in a longer and sudden manner. My head tilted to the side giving me all of one eye. I winked back. Then she winked with her other eye; another clear bold wink just like its twin. I responded in turn with my opposite eye but my attempt was sloppy and spilled all over my face. That was when I realized I was a right-eyed winker.

Conversations in the room muffled. Every sound muted as if it was strained through fine linen. The room blurred itself and moved to the side giving us plenty of room as if we were on a clay court; two athletes in sport.

Violet returned without the slightest effort. Left wink. Right wink. Left wink. Right wink. *How in the hell does she do that*, I thought.

Stephan and Sovina stopped talking. They looked at me and back at Violet. Spectators.

At first one could barely hear her wink but then it got louder. It was hard to believe that a gesture was able to create such a glorious sound.

[The Wink to Signal a Shared Secret:
inspired from the story of Odin the Norse god.
Odin gave his eye in exchange for a drink from
the well of Mimir; a drink which would give him
the gift of great wisdom and knowledge.]

Oh lord I thought. Listen to her. I was learning to distrust the thievery of the dementias. It may sound absurd to say this but there was a kind of glory that she owned at that moment. She was awakening all kinds of thrilling vibrations in her senses drawing me deeper inside. Neighboring patrons heard the winking and looked over to where we were sitting as if we had gone crazy.

"Psst. What's she doing? Over there."

"Is she deaf or something?"

Soon more patrons joined the sport of right-side, left-side winking. Old men shifted their hairy noses from side to side trying to master their serve. Right wink. Left wink. Wrinkled faces, contorted mouths, dentures lifted and dropped in the wink's wave. The room got quiet in surfaced conversations and loud in winks. It was an extraordinary and delightful experience, for which I cannot explain.

A waitress with a large tray balanced on her shoulder, placed a platter of dumplings on the table and covered the clayed court.

34.
COME WITH ME

[In her pocket, Violet found a key
to a gate that when opened would lead her
to everything mysterious and wonderful.
After turning the key in its lock, she gave
the key to her daughter in hopes
that she would join her.]

There were moments when Violet would be confused, then serious and in a second flip her thoughts upside down and laugh. Sometimes she would slip into empty places and settle there for a spell, then pop out through the cracks in its wall and come back to visit. Conversations with sentences properly connected were at a minimum. We all tried to follow but it was as if she snapped her words in two making them meaningless and foreign. She spoke gibberish fluently as if it were her born language.

Her thoughts might have been scattered and unclear but she had pirate eyes; eyes bluer and brighter than any eyes I had ever seen on anyone. They were bright, moist and watered in Caribbean blue pools of unspoken clarity. Pictured memories would float in and out of the yeasty ocean, bumping into each other. Sea urchins full of stories and mysteries waited for any courageous soul to dive in its deep pool. Angelfishes dangled a seductive lure in hope to catch me off my guard. Violet was the long lost queen of these waters.

*

My mother cupped her hand and scooped up the air between us; the directional gesture for a body to come closer. Her eyes held on to me and wouldn't let go. So much seductive magic is at the window's eye. I believed my mother's eyes, her new dementia eyes gave her special powers as well as being the keeper of secrets. But I too had secrets. Her eyes often scared me.

I moved closer to her bed and sat on its mattress edge.

"Come with me." The first spoken words I had heard from my mother in weeks. She talked plainly as in the voice of a woman much younger than herself and more confident.

The room grew smaller and stilled itself. Maybe I didn't hear her correctly. I felt ice on my feet's bare skin and on my back. Her question came at me so quickly and vanished as hurriedly as it came into the air. Behind her all had fallen into silence, waiting for my answer.

My head was stuffed with no sound - the loud and noiseless remains when everything around you stops and your brain is being sent signals that it is hearing something that isn't there. It is a very low hum, an electro-chemical sound of energy that often resonates inside my skull, audible to only my ears when given sufficient quiet.

My mother extended her hands out to mine and held them gently. I pulled them back into myself. "Come with me" she repeated.

I was confused and moved. Did she just ask me to come with her to die? A part of me found her invitation extraordinary yet somewhat inviting. She kept looking at me waiting for an answer. In her eyes I saw a thousand stars against a dark sky. She took me to places that were dark and twisted and turned in unexpected places traveling past the moon, past the galaxy. This fragile woman did not see a daughter, an artist, a visiting young woman with colored hair and paint on her cloths. She was looking at someone bigger, someone inside of me, whom I barely dared to know myself. That is when I had become aware of a negative and ignoble character inside me. I had come face-to-face with my darkest side and at the same time, an extraordinary brilliancy that was all mine. It was terrifying. Outside the windows, you could hear the tired night beat like a napping heart. The curtains breathed in and out. One by one the airheads began to wave quietly in the window's breeze.

"Come with me." She repeated her request that drew me deeper into her follies.

“Eh? Come on now, what would happen to Lil'Vi if I left and went with you?” My senses got the best of me. “You know mom, we can't just both leave her. It would break her heart in two. She'd have a nervous breakdown for sure and end up in some crazy house... you know how sensitive and nervous she is. And Mira, what about Mira? She can't lose a mother and a sister at the same time. No. It would be bad, mom."

After a short pause, I repeated my mind's good sense. “No. That's a bad idea.”

"Oh... Lil'Vi. Yes. She does take everything extra hard.” I was surprised the night summoned her daughters. Did she actually remember she had three daughters?

She concluded, “Maybe you should stay."

We sat close together, without talking, without the sundown gypsies, without MetLife on the TV.

“You look like you've been picking dandelions.”

We both laughed.

She hadn't spoke for months following that day.

35.
THE GIRL WITH TWO BIRTHDAYS

I climbed into my mother's bed and lowered my body as not to be horizontally taller. My head tucked itself into her neck. I shifted my restlessness and straightened my legs against her blanketed bones. Her body was thin and frail. Her toes were curled as if she was standing on the edge of a cliff.

My mother gently touched my cheek. Her hands were arthritically clasped together. Hands she used to fight the demons in the night.

"Mom do you want to hear the Good Friday story - the one about the day the little girl died and came back to life? I can tell you the story and if you want to add something you can."

Silence.

To ease my mother's search for an answer I began the story without her blessing. It was my story even though I had no recollection of being part of any of it. It was simply a great story.

"Ok then, let me start. It's a story about a girl who had two birthdays. Her first birthday was on a warm Chicago day in June and her second birthday was on snowy Good Friday when she was a little girl lying on the floor at Pulaski's Drugstore four years later."

Every Good Friday for as long as I could remember, my mother would tell me about the day I died and came back to life. I heard the story again and again and each time I listened as if I was hearing it for the first time. The story never changed except in the past few years. The story was repeated beyond its Good Friday anniversary date and within its frequent repetitions, the facts got a bit jumbled. Mom added quite a few more characters, television celebrities and dead people, as well as a goat from Indiana and a side trip to Miami Beach for a Tupperware convention. The story took on a kind of fairy-tale-folk-sci-fi-drama genre. I had to use all my brains to follow but the ending was always the same. The little girl lived. My mother stopped telling the story months ago.

The story cleared the room of everything worldly. The balloons of Kitty and Dora floated closer as not to miss any of the good parts.

My mother's Good-Friday-voice could be heard in my head - a voice from years ago. It was stronger and not forgetful. The younger mother started telling the story...

*

"Your father was at work, the day shift at Western Electric. I was upset that he was working on the most religious of holy days. It was snowing heavy, God's punishment to all the weather complaining peoples in Chicago who were at work instead of church. It was the heavy snow that stopped all traffic on the side streets. On the busy streets, cars drove in tunnels made from the snowplows burying the parked cars on each side."

"I was busy in the kitchen wiping down the table from the breakfast morning goop. Mira, your older sister, was in the bathroom straddling the edge of the porcelain tub. One leg was in the tub and the other tapping hard and loud on the bathroom floor. I heard her tappin' all the way in the kitchen. She would tell you to hurry up. Your poop was moving too slow for her."

I don't exactly remember the details. The image had been refined and tailored every time I heard the story: my sister would prop up her head with her fist and with a whole lot of attitude, rest her fist and full arm on one knee – the other leg she used for tapping. Mira was ten, tall for her age and a bit more grown up for just being ten. She had far better things to do than to watch her sister sit on a potty waiting to be intestinally inspired. Serious potty-butt dents or poop would be the only outcome that could end all her suffering.

I remembered the bathroom was small and narrow. On one side of the room was the tub - the other side had the servicing fixtures and hamper. The potty was between the porcelains, the sink and the grounded toilet. The floor was linoleumed with small black and white octagons. Turquoise plastic tiles never completed their climb up the wall. They stopped three quarters of the way. At the far end was an old wood window that opened unevenly. Its lopsided opening made the way for bad air to leave and good air to come inside. Not sure how the airs figured this out but they did and it worked.

I was small for my age and too short to use the room's grown-up toilet. I sat on my own little wooden throne, sitting between the porcelains, resting my crossed arms on my bruised knees, picking at the over-done scabs. I had tree climbing, kick-ass legs for a four year old, filled with bruises and an assortment of black-n-blue moons. The hairs on my head split, creating two cockeyed pigtails above the ears, one considerably higher than another. They evened themselves out when I tilted my head to one side, while sending telepathic messages to my sister Mira - *Don't even think of leaving this room until I poop.* I was sadistic at four.

*

My head helped my mother tell the story, but even in her silence she shoved my words to the side and continued her soundless dialogue.

"Well, you were in the bathroom on the potty and Mira was watching you. And then I heard your sister's a screaming. You know, normally she's not much of a screamer so I go running into the bathroom. She's screaming... *Mom, Suzka is acting crazy, she's shaking all over, come quick, hurry!* Well, when I got there, you were shaking alright like the devil himself was inside of you."

"I didn't know what to think. You were shaking and burning up with the fire's heat. Your cries were stuck inside of you trying to push their way out. You curled your fists around the heat of your fever."

"I grabbed you so fast, bent you over the sink, and let the cold faucet pour its water all over you. At the same time, I yelled over to Mira to turn on the tub water. I told her to use the cold knob only and put in the stopper. Your sister was frozen in place. I had to yell at her again... *Mira, now! Do it now!* I screamed the scare out of her so hard that she back-slammed her body right into the wall. Then she did what I told her to do."

"I ran back into the kitchen to get some ice. I held you tight in one arm. Your face was burning hot. Your whole body was dripping red and still shaking like a mad dog. I don't know how I did it, but in one arm I grabbed everything out of the freezer; ice trays, roasts, frozen peas, everything freezing cold that I could hold. I was scared the fire inside of you would boil your brains."

"I ran back to the bathroom and saw Mira leaning over the tub, lookin' at the faucet, beggin' the water to move quicker. I screamed to her, *Move over, move Mira, move, move, move*. Then I laid you in the tub with one arm and dropped the frozen cold all around you. There was only a little under four inches of water in the tub. You were looking bad. Your eyeballs were rolling all over the place. I had to think with all my brains. Your sister kept asking me if you're gonna die?"

"I then picked you up and ran out into the dining room. I grabbed my coat and laid it flat down on the table and wrapped you up in it. I knew I had to go outside and get some help. I hated to leave Mira alone but I had no choice. I told her not to go anywhere. Don't answer the door, don't answer the phone, don't speak - don't move. That's no good to leave a little one all alone on such a terrible cold day but I had to do it. I had to find help."

"She listened - she listened too much. Mira didn't move - she didn't even go to pee. When I got home, she was exactly where I left her. Your sister was frozen stuck."

I was the teller of the story and the listener at the same time remembering my mother's words and picturing it in my head. After Violet gave Mira the kid-alone-at-home instructions, I saw my mother make twenty *sign-of-the-cross*'s and then run out the door like a shot out of hell. She never included that part in her story telling but I saw it anyway.

The room was quiet. I was lying so close to her I could feel her heartbeat with mine. I couldn't move - my eyes were closed. Without a sound, without a word, my mother's younger voice continued the story...

"I ran down the middle of the street with you in my arms, wearing just a cotton dress and my slippers. I didn't feel the cold at all. You hardly weighed anything. There was a pharmacy a couple of blocks away. I remembered they had a doctor's office on the second floor. I ran down the middle of street as fast as I could, then into the pharmacy and up the side stairs."

"The second floor was dark and had a long hallway of doors on both sides; doors with gold letters on those fancy pitted windows. My eyes were serious. They took me from one door to another looking for the word 'Doctor' on the glass. I was nearly to the end of that hall and I saw, 'Dr. Yurka'. Relief sweat out of my head... but not for long. I couldn't get the door to open. I looked around me - his door, every door was closed, dark window closed. No one was working. It was a holy day. Even good Jewish doctors don't work on Good Friday back then. I walked back down into the pharmacy. I just stood there in place, I couldn't move no more. The cold talked to my head and it started me shaking."

"*My baby's dead,* I said. Everyone looked at me. My hair was crying down my face, my dress was dripping cold water. I was standing there in a puddle of disbelief. I was a mess. *My baby's dead,* I said."

"The pharmacist stopped his pharmacy'ing and ran to me. He took you from my arms and laid you on the floor. When he opened the coat, you were already blue, dead blue, Granpa blue. The skin on your face tinged and your small eyes turned inwards. People in the store were looking down at you and whispering words they sent to the heavens. Everything inside of me left. God took me from all happiness. I thought for sure God had punished me for something I did, something big. Then two firemen walked in like they were the archangels themselves. They came from nowhere. We all moved aside. They knelt over you and brought you out of death and back to the living."

Violet would pause at this part, take a deep breath and change the tone in her voice, taking a more pragmatic approach to end her story.

"Your father came home from work, Mira got unfrozen and I watched over you for two days straight, so the devil wouldn't take you back to convulsions. Everything was back to normal, except you were not the same. You changed. You were like a jumping bean. You could not be still for a minute. It was like you had ants-in-your-pants... and you made me crazy from that day on. Never knew what to expect from you. I talked with God, God talked with the druggist. It was about that time when I started taking the Nervine pills for my nerves. It all worked out. And never again, on Good Friday, did your father go to work.

[There was talk among the family women
that life took away that precious angel from this earth
and dropped in a rather capricious child.]

*

I fell asleep with my head tucked into my mother's neck. The warmth of her body and the rolling wave of her breath immersed me into the warm waters before time.

A sound had swelled in the heat. A muffled sound that started in the corner of the room and grew as it moved closer. I stretched my ears as far as they would go to hear the sound - a run of woods tapping against the steel rims of drums. As the woods got louder the energy intensified. My head was filled with voices that must have come from the moon's side where dreams are painted and filmed. The air around me pulsated and came alive. An impatient curiosity overcame me. I opened my eyes inside my sleep.

The streets were lined with massive crowds. Everyone was dressed in costume and had painted their faces. Plum feathered guards with brassy instruments led to what looked like a parade. Nothing appeared to be what it should be as they do in most dreams.

Everyone was singing, cheering and bumping into each other. They moved like toys wound too tight. Street dancers turned in circles and the birds above flew backwards to confuse the gods. I watched a moving line of cars kiss each other like dogs do when they meet other dogs.

The parade carried on for blocks. Hearses that dropped their tops carried mounds of flowers and wreaths. Cars followed behind with flags on their noses and arms waving out their sides. Some cars had ballooned angels on top with wings so large that if the wind had a mind to, it could blow them away. Saintly characters stuck out of limos' roofs. The likenesses to Michael, Christopher and Jude - they threw wrapped candies into the crowds below. Women in white choir cottons carried ornate offerings on their heads. Other women wore large hooped earrings and charm bracelets with hanging gold amulets. Their blouses were ruffled along the top stretching from shoulder to shoulder. The ruffles lowered themselves seductively showing ample cleavage to the crowd. Their shadows moved like spatters of paint along the streets catching the light as they passed by. The sight was truly spectacular. The energy was intoxicating. The smell was hot and moist with human perspiration that lodged in my nose and my throat. I swallowed the night's dream and started counting the cars in the procession. "Forty-seven, forty-eight, forty-nine, fifty..." In the distance, down the long street a Virgin'd statue paled.

I walked along the curb and followed the parade to a city's circle where an improvised altar was built. It was curtained in gold beaded fabric and cornered with bouquets of jasmine.

In front of the altar was a large cauldron filled with paper scribbled notes folded three or four times. The notes contained offerings, memories people would give to the gods in exchange for true happiness. The music and cheering intensified. The crowds compressed. Waving arms with fists clutching their papered memories squeezed and pushed their way to the cauldron where they would place their offerings. After much anticipation and quite suddenly, fire-eaters from the parade took their torches and lit the caldron on fire. I had my back turned and it wasn't until the cauldron and the altar was engulfed in flames did I realize what had taking place. Smoke and ashes flew into the air and fell down on us like feathered snow, baby feathers from a young chic.

One of the performers broke out of the parade and walked toward me. My body contracted with a shot of feelings. He saw the troubled look in my eyes, a look like I should not be there. He was not an old man and not a young boy. He sat in the middle of deciding. On his head was a black top hat.

The kindly boy-man walked straight to me and when he got quite close, he swept the top hat off his head and bowed. His voice came out big like his presence. His head leveled to my eyes and asked. "Come with us. Come join the parade."

A moon woke me up.

< UNITED AIRLINES >

DEPART: Chicago

ARRIVE: California

EXPIRED

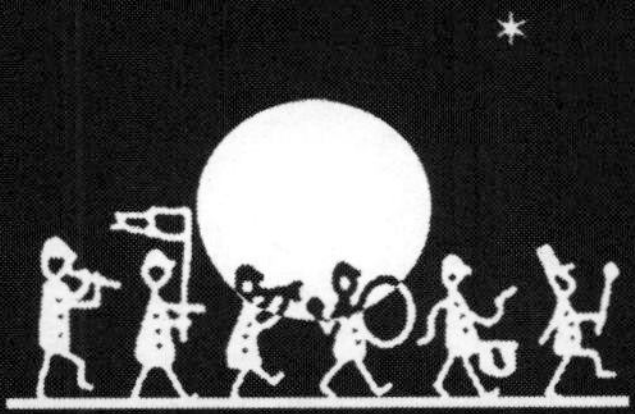

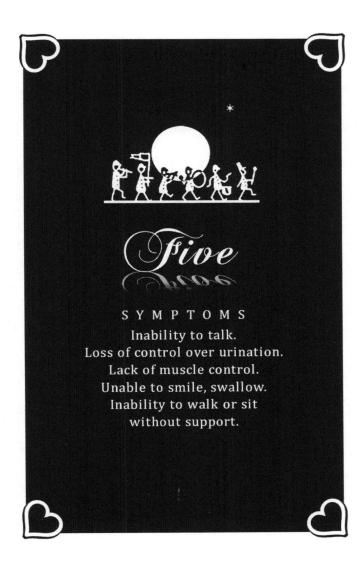

Five

SYMPTOMS

Inability to talk.
Loss of control over urination.
Lack of muscle control.
Unable to smile, swallow.
Inability to walk or sit
without support.

[I thought this all had to end sometime.
And then it did.]

36.
SHE'S READY

Sovina ran downstairs to call for me. She grabbed me out of a dead sleep. I followed behind her back up the stairs. I couldn't hear myself running but I knew I was because I bumped into the railing corner at the top landing. My bones told me to forget the bruising pain and hurry. I stumbled into the room where my mother lay. A bright light from the moon covered everything. The room inhaled and held me in its breath, as I stood motionless in the center of its silence.

Life broke its fever. They wouldn't come back to help her this time. The doctors, hospice too, told me they would not come back. Her organs were not strong enough to continue their work.

Sovina knew what to do. I could only watch. She peeled away one blanket from my mother and then another. Slowly and with grace she peeled away all her coverings. Outside the stars watched. We all watched.

My mother was as stiff as a broken puppet. Her legs were rigid in place and crooked. I was hoping she would not travel to the next life with crooked legs. Her face was beautiful. Her eyelids looked as if they were carved by the hands of a saint-maker.

I heard the music of my family play in my head. Faraway music. Music coming from parade-ians flanked with banners, fans, silver crosses on long poles and tall candles. Plum feathered guards with brassy instruments played.

"Stephan!" I thought, "Of course, Mom would want to hear Stephan's music for sure. Where in the hell are his CDs. Which one? Which one should I play? The boombox. Where's the boombox?"

I did not recognize my own voice. I ran to the counter and nervously fumbled with Stephan's CD. My hands were shaking and confused. For the life of me, I could not remember how to make that damn cheap box work. Moisture beaded on my forehead. My hand searched my head for help.

Sovina began washing my mother's body, washing away the illness. She didn't want my mother to take her broken brains with her. When she finished, Sovina opened the window telling death, his bride was ready.

Skeeter took Violet's arm. He would take her to her death. "*Are you ready?*" He said to her. "*It is time.*"

She seemed to hesitate as though she was giving her decision to go a second thought.

Violet looked around the room behind her veil. Her new eyes followed a white aisle runner sprinkled with rose petals. At the end, a large thick man stood with a smile so wide it caused his eyes to disappear in its crease. He looked familiar. She squinted and looked closer. His hair was white as snow. He dressed in a gray suit with purple Violets pinned to its lapel. He was there to officiate something. Violet was unclear but resigned and was comforted by his presence. The large man thought her beautiful. He nodded - the nod a father would give to a daughter as a sign of approval. Standing to the left side of the officiator was her groom, her death, dressed like an admiral. He wore a white dress suit gilded in bands of cadmium and plates of gold. Aiguillettes laced across his chest. His heart was covered with shiny stars, precious jewels and gold-laced buttons. Violet could hardly breathe in anticipation.

The bells rang quietly throughout the house - they had no stones in them. The trees outside looked in the windows and rustled with excitement.

Violet peeked out from behind a vestibule window and counted the receiving guests... *fifty six, fifty seven, fifty eight...*

Softly, Violet closed her eyes.

My body folded as though someone shot a bullet into my bones.

Slowly I bent over death and kissed my mother's cheek. It was cold and felt like wax paper. She smelled clean and dry like a scoured plate.

Something pushed me back, away from death's draft. I dug my feet as deep as I could into the living side of the room and tightened my jaw. I didn't want to be swallowed into the bowels of the devil. He could be here too. I was not always a good girl and wasn't about to take any chances.

I looked at the bed where life once lay. Violet's hands were crossed and rested quietly above her cotton nightgown. She was covered in white with a wonderful face.

Death lifted life's veil and kissed my mother before us.

The music crescendo'ed - everything was louder, the sound of passage, the volume, the intensity increased. Stephan fiercely pounded on the piano keys inside the boombox - Liszt's Liebestraum No.3.

The gypsies danced faster and harder as though they were caught in a typhoon. Their colors circled around and through the wedding guests. Older gypsy women with sunken eyes and loose teeth bounced up and down on their weathered bare feet with leathered bottoms; the callused sign of centuries of dancing. They carried cloth brocade bags. From their bags they dug deep and grabbed a handful of stolen memories and sprinkled them around the room like wedding confetti.

The balloons of Cookie, Kitty, Betty Boop, Belle and Dora shook, scat and shimmied. The other airheads bounced and pulled on their ribbons scooting their weighted hearts around the room. Their feet moved wickedly over the carpet, the sound of their mouths spoke not a word joyously.

Violet's face paled and reflected the faces of the dead passing through a mirror; faces of loved ones who traveled far to be here for the celebration. The walls opened letting them in. They brought with them the sweet aromas of calla lilies, violets, roses and jasmine.

Then all at once, the sainted statues throughout the house came to life - the Madonnas and Jesuses, the Michaels and the Christophers – all the consecrated creatures that nourished my family's restlessness for decades, as the earth, the sun and the skies could not, they all came to see my mother. The blessed statues wiggled and twisted their bodies loose from their footings and squirmed out of their plaster molds. Once freed, they rushed into death's room. Their gowns, their cloaks flapped behind them making a sound like the hands of clapping madmen. They would welcome the guested ghosts who were waiting to greet the bride, drink wine and resurrect their connections.

Picasso, Giacometti and Gulley were not there. They were not invited or just busy.

My mother accepted death's dance. She had no pulse or will. She had committed herself. Her young legs moved around the dance floor to the music played. She waved at the guests who watched her. She was light on her feet and spun around the room. Death tightly held her in his arms like any loving groom would. Violet danced breathlessly with her distinguished partner. The moon and the stars circled and swayed back and forth to Stephan's lover's dream music playing in the boombox faraway. For blocks away the noise and music could not be heard, neighbors would not complain.

Once death took Violet's hand, she left the party. The shyness of it, the almost frightened way she followed was daunting. They walked together into a small adjoining room. There she sat on the pillowed bed of her commitment. She took off her veil, placed it in on her lap and crossed her hands laying them delicately on the white netting. On the wall was a picture of her three children, a family portrait. Her eyes remembered.

She kicked off her shoes. Death removed his jacket and loosened his shirt. His face was summered in moonlight blue. He laughed loudly taking her life into his belly. Her tiny body moved in and out of life. Death then shut its door. Their bond was consummated.

Life had packed its time readying itself to move on.

*

The shuffling noise of the crowd's feet left the room. The balloons barely moved. They wanted to wave goodbye but couldn't. The cold air blew the white curtains gently away from the window. The music ceased. There was a voice talking in my head that never finished its thought. The moon was dimming in its light from the sun pushing it aside.

My mother's body jerked hard – after-death spasms. The Miss America tiara fell from the corner head-frame of the bed. The sky held tightly on to its moon so it wouldn't fall.

I stared at my mother for a long time. I thought I saw her look up once. Death was playing tricks on me. My eyes kept fixed until I could not recognize her face.

Someone shook my world upside down and shook my family out. I felt genocide's emptiness. I had nowhere to go. California, my warehouse, all my colors moved to another planet outside this galaxy. I wondered if my life would remember who I was. It's been close to three years. That's a long time to leave a life on its own. And my ghostly mentors, we haven't spoken for such a very long time. Maybe they all moved away without telling me. The air was cold. Everything had changed so fast. I was empty.

Sovina went into the kitchen to prepare the foods for the expected guests. She looked into the cabinets for altar wine and wedding champagne. Stephan and Tony and for sure Rosetta would be arriving soon.

[Rosetta was the family's personal mortician.]

37.
AFTER ROSETTA

I raised every bottle to the light, checking the fluid levels looking for old champagne or altar wine that stayed the night. The boombox was still playing

Stephan's music. Stephan left hours earlier, just after the mortician took my mother away. Everyone had left. Sovina went to her room.

It was late. Yesterday was hanging around a bit longer. The windows finished creating reflections of the tired guests and reversing them on its glass; mirrored images that magically showed the other side of things.

Kitty, Dora, Belle and a few others kept to themselves comforting each other. Yawns could have separated their conversations. I was disinterested in kibitzing. It was over. My imagination had lost all its social graces.

I leaned over the small round table in the far corner of the room. One bottle with a visible promising liquid line caught my attention. It was sitting between a few broken cabbage horns and warped salami slices. Chunks of hardened baguettes lumped around the hardened treats. A few crusts fell into a bowl where two bruised strawberries sat on the bottom, looking bloody and defeated. Nothing was put away or fridg'ed.

My reach for the bottle hung the edge of my blouse over the table, licking the puffed cream off of the food gummed plates in its way. I collected just enough champagne from a few opened bottles to fill one glass to its half. The bubbles were gone and the liquid was flat. Champagne bubbles are always the first to leave a party.

Ripped apart from the day, I pulled a chair out, away from the small table and slumped down. I felt a kick in my stomach that would paralyze an elephant. *Where did everything go? What had happened to me?*

I was already missing some sense of my self. I lived in Dementialand for so long that I was getting quite comfortable in the vast openness of its own reality - the craziness and confusion, the gibberish, the anger and the final surrender of it all - surrendering to the place where I was able to see for miles without the yesterdays and tomorrows obstructing my view. It was difficult and so simple all at the same time.

The mirrors of dementia showed me the reverse-ness of its doings. Mirrors and the night's glass windows understood. They reflected the other side of everything - the other side of myself.

I saw my mother with eyes opened and not curtained by her motherhood or my ego. And when I finally listened, really listened, I found my 'self'. My mother and I became part owners of each other, engaged in growing away from who we thought we were suppose to be.

But where was I to go from here? The pervasiveness of dementia's cock-eyed reality was closing its opening. I was unplugged from the outside world. The thought of going back to a world I outgrew was scary.

Oh shut up already! All this thinking, all these thoughts running in and out of my head – all this worry is gonna give me a bigger headache than the one I already have. Maybe I should eat something - put something solid in my stomach to soak up the liquid remains of this night.

I started looking for breakfast possibilities. As a rule, I never ate breakfast. The egg-toast-fruit combination was a delicacy I only savored after a long night of drinking and dancing. For me breakfast was a chaser.

But I was feeling emptied. My mouth was pasted with the remains of yesterday; my stomach felt like a rabid mad dog - a crust of bread, a chip, a pretzel, would help.

Leaning back in the chair and pushing my feet out, I stretched my neck back as far as it would go. Maybe bending my bones would improve the circulation in my head and in the room. As I looked up I noticed there was a broken glass from a fixture hanging above the table. It wasn't hard to miss. I vaguely remembered a cork going off at sometime, shattering the light's glass shade. The bulb inside was miraculously unharmed. It appeared to be a clean cork shot.

I looked around the room. There must have been ten or twelve large balloons scattered around - balloons with those stupid painted faces. Cinderella, Snow White and the Cookie Monster, Tweety-Bird and Sponge Bob, they all seemed to be looking directly at me with such benevolence.

"Now what?" I asked.

I turned my words to the group, Kitty, Betty and Dora. They were clustered close together as if they were in a gossipy conversation. Their ballooned heads stood around lazy-like and turned softly toward the broken fixture. I picked up my slump from the chair and quasi-questioned the group. "What are you looking at? Did anyone of you see what happened here? Any witnesses who have something to say?" The balloons, almost in unison, spoke to my exhausted imagination.

"I didn't see anything'."

"No, not me, I saw nothing."

"I wasn't here, I was with Kitty."

"Anyone else got something not-to-say?"

Looking up at the fixture, I thought of how pissed my mother would have been. Mom loved that light fixture. *"Suzka, I told you to go out on the porch and point that loaded bottle outside when you're popping it. You're gonna break a window in here or shoot the head off of Jesus, God help us."*

I looked over to the other side of the room where the life size Jesus stood. Thank God, He was looking good - no battle wounds.

I found a big chunk of glass lying on the cabbage horns' platter. Rosetta earlier took a full plate of the pastries home for her father. Hopefully, there weren't any glass shavings in her sugared selections. You don't want to get on the bad side of Rosetta.

Rosetta was the family's personal mortician - a lady in her forties with a go-get-um personality and a stack of calendars; business calendars, showing twelve different religious scenes on the top half of each open page and boxed days of the month on the bottom half. In big bold letters, 'Hudak Funeral Services' was visible on each page. Punched holes were centered on the top for nail hanging. Everyone in the family had a Hudak calendar displayed somewhere in their home.

Rosetta does everyone in the family, sooner or later. It's been that way for decades. Her father was a mortician; his father was a mortician; his father's father... and so on. Now his daughter, Rosetta, handles all the family business. It would be unheard-of, somewhat sacrilegious, grossly irreverent and simply too risky to have any other mortician drain and dress a loved one, other than Rosetta.

Loyalties to Rosetta were well earned. She was good. She had a way of putting the tiniest little smile on her body's faces. They all had that look - the look a body has when they're telling you, without a word spoken, *I know exactly what you've done, what you said and where you hid the bodies.* She was a master.

My mother's voice hung on my ear like a clip-on earring, irritatingly pinching the skin. *"Did you give Rosetta any candy? Remember to give her an extra bag of the sugarless for her father. He's diabetic. Don't fill the bag. I don't want to cause any more bad luck now that his wife died."*

I drifted around in my thoughts and eventually fell asleep. Hours later, the back porch door slammed shut and woke me up. My mother hadn't followed all the rules of death. She had walked out into the new morning to feed the birds for the last time.

[I made peace with dementia and
thanked its gods for their gift.
I learned to talk to mermaids,
dance with the gypsies and smell
the flowering jasmines in front of me.
As for my mother, who remained
untouched in details, her dementia
nourished life's perplexing quandary
and returned her to her 'self'.]

38.
MOVING JESUS

"Over here. It's pretty heavy... I'm not sure how you're going to do this... You'll have to wrap him up good with some thick bubble-wrap and padded blankets... use everything you got."

They followed me, two men, two big men in blue muscled uniforms. "There He is."

"That's a... Jesus. Holy crap."

"I know. I told your moving company about it... about Him. He's big."

"I never moved a Jesus before. Is He for real? I mean..." The mover man tapped hard with one finger on the side of Jesus's shoulder. "Oh my God, He is the real thing. This is solid plaster. He must weigh a ton."

The mover man squeezed his face, wiped his hands on his pant leg and yelled over his shoulder. "Hey Frank, you better bring in the refrigerator dolly." Frank was outside by the truck and heard him clearly.

"Just be careful and wrap him tightly. Don't want him to lose his head or any of his fingers...God forbid."

"Where's he goin'? In a church or somethin'?"

"No. He's moving in with me... in California... in my studio."

It took three solid thick men to move Jesus. They wrapped Him tightly in heavy padding. Then two men tilted the weight forward. The other man slid the dolly's lip under Jesus. Thick rubber straps tightened everything in place. Jesus's head stuck out of the padding. The wheels made it around the corner. At first all you heard was the dolly crack and heave on its wooden joints. The men stumbled carefully down each step holding onto the plastered weight of everything deemed blessed. They went into the street to the back of the truck and slowly rolled the dolly with Jesus up a ten-foot metal plank that rested on the truck's edge.

The men's faces turned rose colored and then pale. Wet beads of sweat water crossed their foreheads and necks. Jesus's painted face never changed. The men finished wrapping Him tightly and secured His position in the truck for the long trip.

I walked to the curbstone and watched. My eyes moved about the street. The leaves ran around me confused. An old woman looking out her window caught my attention. Maybe she was worried about Jesus's fate. She crossed herself three times and then took a puff from her cigarette. The white smoke curled around her face.

The house was empty. Everything was sold or given away or taken to the Salvation Army. The Got-Junk people picked up the unacceptable items.

Everyone was gone except for Kitty, Betty, Dora and Belle and two Elmo's - the last residents standing in Dementialand. They kept to themselves huddled in one corner their round skins were buffed by the afternoon sun. My airhead friends with no arms and legs quivered a bit. They all seemed to be looking at me. Kitty was in front and barely moved.

I gathered the group, clutched their ribboned strings in my hand and walked outside. Their metal weighted hearts dragged behind. They softly rustled against each other in excitement. The sun sparkled down on them hard like crushed pearls. I leaned over the porch's ledge and raised my ribboned hand over the rail, looking up to where I was cutting the strings of the balloons. Then in one swift cut the balloons left me like white birds. I watched them leave me. They ran to a small hole in the sky and disappeared. My eyes got brittle from staring into the brightness.

*

"Jaidee?"

"Yes dis iz Jaidee."

"This is Suzka.."

"Miz Suzka. It has been so long since..."

"Can you please come and get me?"

< UNITED AIRLINES >

FLIGHT: #841 Fri Dec11

DEPART: Chicago at 9:55 AM

ARRIVE: California at 3:57 PM

ONE-WAY

EPILOGUE

I forgot to count the cars in my mother's funeral procession. She later came to me in a dream and told me she counted fifty-nine.

DEMENTIALAND CHARACTERS

Dementialand's Main Characters:

- *Violet: mother, Slovakian matriarch of her family living in Chicago*
- *Suzka: daughter, artist, moved to Chicago from California to care for Violet*
- *Pavel: Violet's husband, died eight years prior to Violet's illness*
- *Lil'Vi: Violet's younger daughter*
- *Mira: Violet's older daughter*
- *Jaidee: limo driver and friend of Suzka*
- *Sovina: caregiver living with Violet and Suzka*
- *Ellie: Violet's church friend*
- *Billy: visiting nurse*
- *Rosetta: family mortician*

Illusionary Characters - large faced balloons

- *Cookie: (male) the first balloon*
- *Hello Kitty: likeness to a levelheaded, sophisticated woman about thirty, thirty five*
- *Princess Belle: likeness to a cross dressing Mexican sweetheart*
- *Dora: likeness to a black woman from Gary Indiana, smart, not afraid of nottin', an ebony temptress*
- *Smilie: always happy, lives in the moment*
- *Twins Elmos: likenesses to Bostonian jokesters. Blue Elmo is open, thinks outside the box; Red Elmo follows the rules, conservative*

additional balloons - no speaking roles:

- *Nemo, Sleeping Beauty, Little Mermaid, Sponge Bob, Betty Boop, Tweedy Bird, Cinderella, Snow White and Big Bird, butterflies, stars, hearts*

Delusional Characters:

- *Skeeter is 'dementia', full name, Anopheles de'Mantia*
- *Gypsy dancers*
- *Statue'd Saints*

DEMENTIA
IS NOT A DISEASE

Dementia is not a specific disease. It's an overall term that describes a wide range of symptoms associated with a decline in memory or other thinking skills severe enough to reduce a person's ability to perform everyday activities.

People with dementia may have problems with short-term memory, keeping track of a purse or wallet, paying bills, planning and preparing meals, remembering appointments or traveling out of the neighborhood. While symptoms of dementia can vary greatly, at least two of the following core mental functions must be significantly impaired to be considered dementia: memory, communication and language, ability to focus and pay attention, reasoning and judgment and visual perception. Many dementias are progressive, meaning symptoms start out slowly and gradually get worse.

Alzheimer's disease accounts for 60 to 80 percent of cases. Vascular dementia, which occurs after a stroke, is the second most common dementia type. Lewy Bodies Dementia changes the way muscles work and mimics Parkinson's disease.

*

CASE: <u>Alzheimer's disease</u>

Alzheimer's disease accounts for up to 50% to 70% of cases of dementia.

Alzheimer symptoms:

In the early stages of Alzheimer's disease, patients may experience memory impairment, lapses of judgment, and subtle changes in personality. As the disorder progresses, memory and language problems worsen and patients begin to have difficulty performing activities of daily living, such as balancing a checkbook or remembering to take medications. They also may have visuospatial problems, such as difficulty navigating an unfamiliar route. They may become disoriented about places and times, may suffer delusions (such as the idea that someone is stealing from them or that their spouse is being unfaithful) and may become short-tempered and hostile. During the late stages of the disease, patients begin to lose the ability to control motor functions. They may have difficulty swallowing and lose bowel and bladder control. They eventually lose the ability to recognize family members and to speak. As Alzheimer's disease progresses, it begins to affect the person's emotions and behavior. Most people with Alzheimer's disease eventually develop symptoms such as aggression, agitation, depression, sleeplessness, or delusions.

Alzheimer brain changes:

Alzheimer's disease is characterized by two abnormalities in the brain: amyloid plaques and neurofibrillary tangles. Amyloid plaques, which are found in the tissue between the nerve cells, are unusual clumps of a protein called beta amyloid along with degenerating bits of neurons and other cells.

Neurofibrillary tangles are bundles of twisted filaments found within neurons. These tangles are largely made up of a protein called tau. In healthy neurons, the tau protein helps the functioning of microtubules, which are part of the cell's structural support and deliver substances throughout the nerve cell. However, in Alzheimer's disease, tau is changed in a way that causes it to twist into pairs of helical filaments that collect into tangles. When this happens, the microtubules cannot function correctly and they disintegrate. This collapse of the neuron's transport system may impair communication between nerve cells and cause them to die.

CASE: Vascular dementia

Previously known as multi-infarct or post-stroke dementia, vascular dementia is the second most common cause of dementia, after Alzheimer's disease. It accounts for up to 20 percent of all dementia cases.

Vascular dementia symptoms:

Vascular dementia often begins suddenly, frequently after a stroke. Patients may have a history of high blood pressure, vascular disease, or previous strokes or heart attacks. Vascular dementia may or may not get worse with time, depending on whether the person has additional strokes. In some cases, symptoms may get better with time. When the disease does get worse, it often progresses in a stepwise manner, with sudden changes in ability. Vascular dementia with brain damage to the mid-brain regions, however, may cause a gradual, progressive cognitive impairment that may look much like Alzheimer's disease. Unlike people with Alzheimer's disease, people with vascular dementia often maintain their personality and normal levels of emotional responsiveness until the later stages of the disease.

Vascular dementia brain changes:

Vascular dementia is caused by brain damage from cerebrovascular or cardiovascular problems - usually strokes. It also may result from genetic diseases, endocarditis (infection of a heart valve), or amyloid angiopathy (a process in which amyloid protein builds up in the brain's blood vessels, sometimes causing hemorrhagic or "bleeding" strokes).

There are several types of vascular dementia, which vary slightly in their causes and symptoms. One type, called multi-infarct dementia (MID), is caused by numerous small strokes in the brain. MID typically includes multiple damaged areas, called infarcts, along with extensive lesions in the white matter, or nerve fibers, of the brain

CASE: Lewy Bodies Dementia

Lewy body dementia is one of the most common types of progressive dementia. Lewy bodies was first recognized as a diagnosis in the 1980s. Because the signs and symptoms of Lewy bodies dementia resemble those of other forms of dementia, researchers think that the number of diagnoses is lower than the number of cases that actually exist. Lewy bodies are often found in the brains of people with Parkinson Disease. According to the National Institute of Neurological Disorders and Stroke (NINDS), Dementia with Lewy bodies has three features that distinguish it from other forms of dementia: 1.Fluctuating effects on mental functioning, particularly alertness and attention, which may resemble delirium; 2. Recurrent visual hallucinations; and 3. Parkinson-like movement symptoms, such as rigidity and lack of spontaneous movement

Lewy body dementia symptoms:

People with dementia with Lewy bodies often have memory loss and thinking problems common in Alzheimer's, but are more likely than people with Alzheimer's to have initial or early symptoms such as sleep disturbances, well-formed visual hallucinations, and slowness, gait imbalance or other Parkinsonian movement features.

Lewy body dementia brain changes:

In Lewy bodies, cells die in the brain's cortex, or outer layer, and in a part of the mid-brain called the substantia nigra. Many of the remaining nerve cells in the substantia nigra contain abnormal structures called Lewy bodies that are the hallmark of the disease. Lewy bodies may also appear in the brain's cortex, or outer layer. Lewy bodies contain a protein called alpha-synuclein that has been linked to Parkinson's disease and several other disorders.

CASE: <u>Frontotemporal Dementia</u>

Frontotemporal dementia, sometimes called Pick's disease or frontal lobe dementia, describes a group of diseases characterized by the degeneration of nerve cells - especially those in the frontal and temporal lobes of the brain the areas generally associated with personality, behavior and language.

<u>Frontotemporal dementia symptoms</u>:

Because structures found in the frontal and temporal lobes of the brain control judgment and social behavior, people with Frontotemporal dementia often have problems maintaining normal interactions and following social conventions. They may steal or exhibit impolite and socially inappropriate behavior, and they may neglect their normal responsibilities. Other common symptoms include loss of speech and language, compulsive or repetitive behavior, increased appetite, and motor problems such as stiffness and balance problems. Memory loss also may occur, although it typically appears late in the disease.

<u>Frontotemporal dementia brain changes</u>:

Frontotemporal dementia is a result from the shrinking of the outer layers of your brain in the areas just above your eyes (the frontal lobes) and/or close to your ears (the temporal lobes). As the healthy neurons slowly degenerate, they often accumulate abnormally folded proteins.

Other diseases that cause dementia

Parkinson's Disease, Creutzfeldt-Jakob Disease, Normal Pressure Hydrocephalus, Huntington's Disease, Wernicke-Korsakoff Syndrome, Chronic traumatic encephalopathy (CTE), Korsakoff syndrome, Normal Pressure Hydrocephalus, Lyme Disease, Aphasia, Traumatic brain injury and certain viral infections as in Meningitis and Encephalitis.

Dementia Is Not a Disease references:

Alzheimer's Association
http://www.alz.org/dementia/types-of-dementia.asp#dlb
http://www.alz.org/what-is-dementia.asp

Stanford Health Care
https://stanfordhealthcare.org/search-results.html/dementia

National Institute of Neurological Disorders & Stroke
http://www.ninds.nih.gov/disorders/dementias/dementia.htm

Mayo Clinic
http://www.mayoclinic.org/diseases-conditions/dementia/home/ovc-20198502

Science Daily
https://www.sciencedaily.com/news/mind_brain/dementia/

Suzka

Behind the Scenes
A Special Thank You to

Mom

Stuart

Tony, Steve, Paul, Mose,
Lil'Vi and Zita.

Allen, Craig, Chelsea, Ha, Grant,
Gerold, Carol, Michael, Mandy,
Herb, Josh, Olivia,
Michelle, LaLa, Dalena, Rachel,
Sabrina, Ernesto, Trevor,
Carol and Jack, Janet
and Sidney.